T0226820

Peripheral Nerve Disease in the Geriatric Population

Editor

PETER H. JIN

CLINICS IN GERIATRIC MEDICINE

www.geriatric.theclinics.com

May 2021 • Volume 37 • Number 2

ELSEVIER

1600 John F. Kennedy Boulevard • Suite 1800 • Philadelphia, Pennsylvania, 19103-2899

http://www.theclinics.com

CLINICS IN GERIATRIC MEDICINE Volume 37, Number 2
May 2021 ISSN 0749–0690, ISBN-13: 978-0-323-79603-3

Editor: Katerina Heidhausen
Developmental Editor: Ann Posedio

Clinics in Geriatric Medicine (ISSN 0749-0690) is published quarterly by Elsevier Inc., 360 Park Avenue South, New York, NY 10010-1710. Months of issue are February, May, August, and November. Business and Editorial Offices: 1600 John F. Kennedy Blvd., Suite 1800, Philadelphia, PA 191023-2899. Periodicals postage paid at New York, NY, and additional mailing offices. Subscription prices are $295.00 per year (US individuals), $875.00 per year (US institutions), $100.00 per year (US & Canadian student/resident), $320.00 per year (Canadian individuals), $928.00 per year (Canadian institutions), $418.00 per year (international individuals), $928.00 per year (international institutions), and $195.00 per year (international student/resident). Foreign air speed delivery is included in all *Clinics* subscription prices. All prices are subject to change without notice. POSTMASTER: Send address changes to *Clinics in Geriatric Medicine,* Elsevier Health Sciences Division, Subscription Customer Service, 3251 Riverport Lane, Maryland Heights, MO 63043. **Telephone: 1-800-654-2452 (U.S. and Canada); 314-447-8871 (outside U.S. and Canada). Fax: 314-447-8029. E-mail:** journalscustomerservice-usa@elsevier.com **(for print support) or** journalsonlinesupport-usa@elsevier.com **(for online support).**

Reprints. For copies of 100 or more, of articles in this publication, please contact the Commercial Reprints Department, Elsevier Inc., 360 Park Avenue South, New York, New York 10010-1710. Tel.: 212-633-3874; Fax: 212-633-3820, E-mail: reprints@elsevier.com.

Clinics in Geriatric Medicine is covered in *MEDLINE/PubMed (Index Medicus), EMBASE/Excerpta Medica, Current Contents/Clinical Medicine (CC/CM),* and the *Cumulative Index to Nursing & Allied Health Literature.*

Contributors

EDITOR

PETER H. JIN, MD
Assistant Professor, Department of Neurology, University of Maryland School of Medicine, Baltimore, Maryland

AUTHORS

RORY M.C. ABRAMS, MD
Department of Neurology, Division of Neuromuscular Diseases and Clinical Neurophysiology Laboratories, Icahn School of Medicine at Mount Sinai, New York, New York

SUUR BILICILER, MD
Associate Professor, Department of Neurology, The University of Texas Health Science Center at Houston, McGovern Medical School, Houston, Texas

JOSEPH M. CHOI, MD
Assistant Professor of Neurology, Georgetown University, Department of Neurology, MedStar Washington Hospital Center, MedStar Georgetown University Hospital, Washington, DC

STEPHEN ZACHARY COX, DO
Department of Neurology, Virginia Commonwealth University, Richmond, Virginia

GIANLUCA DI MARIA, MD
Neurology Resident, Department of Neurology, MedStar Georgetown University Hospital, Washington, DC

HEINRICH ELINZANO, MD
Associate Professor of Neurology, Alpert Medical School of Brown University, Rhode Island Hospital, Providence, Rhode Island

SVETLANA FAKTOROVICH, MD
Florida Atlantic University, Charles E. Schmidt College of Medicine, Marcus Neuroscience Institute, Boca Raton Regional Hospital, Boca Raton, Florida

ASIA FILATOV, MD
Florida Atlantic University, Charles E. Schmidt College of Medicine, Marcus Neuroscience Institute, Boca Raton Regional Hospital, Boca Raton, Florida

NATALIA L. GONZALEZ, MD
Medical Instructor, Department of Neurology, Neuromuscular Division, Duke University, Duke University Hospital, Durham, North Carolina

ANDRE GRANGER, MD, MBA
Resident Physician, Department of Neurology, NYU Grossman School of Medicine, New York, New York

KELLY G. GWATHMEY, MD
Assistant Professor, Department of Neurology, Virginia Commonwealth University, Richmond, Virginia

LISA D. HOBSON-WEBB, MD
Associate Professor, Department of Neurology, Neuromuscular Division, Duke University, Duke University Hospital, Durham, North Carolina

PETER H. JIN, MD
Assistant Professor, Department of Neurology, University of Maryland School of Medicine, Baltimore, Maryland

JUSTIN KWAN, MD
Associate Research Physician, National Institute of Neurological Disorders and Stroke, National Institutes of Health, Bethesda, Maryland

YAOWAREE LEAVELL, MD
Department of Neurology, Icahn School of Medicine at Mount Sinai, New York, New York

RAJEEV MOTIWALA, MD, FAAN
Clinical Professor, Department of Neurology, NYU Grossman School of Medicine, New York, New York

ELIZABETH J. PEDOWITZ, MD
Brookdale Department of Geriatrics and Palliative Medicine, Icahn School of Medicine at Mount Sinai, New York, New York

ZUFE RIZVI, MD
Florida Atlantic University, Charles E. Schmidt College of Medicine, Marcus Neuroscience Institute, Boca Raton Regional Hospital, Boca Raton, Florida

GEORGE SACHS, MD, PhD
Professor of Neurology, Alpert Medical School of Brown University, Rhode Island Hospital, Providence, Rhode Island

JONATHAN SAREZKY, MD
Alpert Medical School of Brown University, Rhode Island Hospital, Providence, Rhode Island

SUSAN C. SHIN, MD
Department of Neurology, Icahn School of Medicine at Mount Sinai, New York, New York

DAVID M. SIMPSON, MD
Department of Neurology, Division of Neuromuscular Diseases and Clinical Neurophysiology Laboratories, Icahn School of Medicine, New York, New York

KARA STAVROS, MD
Assistant Professor of Neurology, Alpert Medical School of Brown University, Rhode Island Hospital, Providence, Rhode Island

ELINA ZAKIN, MD
Assistant Professor, Department of Neurology, NYU Grossman School of Medicine, New York, New York

LAN ZHOU, MD, PhD
Professor of Neurology and Pathology, Department of Neurology, Director, Boston Medical Center Cutaneous Nerve Laboratory, Boston University School of Medicine, Boston, Massachusetts

LINDSAY A. ZILLIOX, MD, MS
Assistant Professor, Department of Neurology, University of Maryland School of Medicine, Maryland VA Healthcare System, Baltimore, Maryland

Contents

 Video content accompanies this article at http://www.geriatric. theclinics.com.

Peripheral neuropathy is one of the most prevalent neurologic conditions encountered by neurologists and nonneurologists. Geriatricians and primary care physicians often face the task of screening patients for early neuropathy when they have underlying conditions such as diabetes mellitus and evaluating patients who report new symptoms that suggest neuropathy. An understanding about different forms of neuropathies based on anatomic pattern and type of nerve fiber involvement and ability to perform basic neurologic examination reliably can help determine how to pursue further investigations and identify those patients who are likely to benefit from early specialist referral.

Nerve conduction studies and electromyography are useful diagnostic tools that neurologists use to diagnose diseases of the peripheral nerves, neuromuscular junction, and muscles. These tests are considered an extension of clinical history and examination, and their results should always be interpreted with the clinical context. Neuromuscular diseases are common and affect a large proportion of the elderly population. With an aging population in expansion, these diseases are expected to become even more prevalent. It is important to highlight the basics of electrophysiology and provide a reference for providers who are planning to send their patients to electromyographers for these studies.V

Peripheral nerve imaging is a helpful and sometimes essential adjunct to clinical history, physical examination, and electrodiagnostic studies. Advances in imaging technology have allowed the visualization of nerve structures and their surrounding tissues. The clinical applications of ultrasound and magnetic resonance imaging (MRI) in the evaluation of peripheral nerve disorders are growing exponentially. This article reviews basics of ultrasound and MRI as they relate to nerve imaging, reviews advantages and limitations of each imaging modality, reviews the applications of ultrasound and MRI in disorders of peripheral nerve, and discusses emerging advances in the field.

Compression neuropathies, also known as entrapment neuropathies, are common neurologic conditions seen in medicine. These often are due to mechanical injury, either compression or stretch of the affected nerve, and initially result in focal demyelinating changes. If left untreated, secondary axonal injury and lasting disability can result. Patients typically present with pain, sensory changes, and potentially weakness in the distribution of the affected nerve; therefore, a basic knowledge of neuromuscular anatomy is necessary to identify these conditions. Initial treatment of mild to moderate cases often is conservative. In severe cases or those refractory to conservative therapy, surgery should be considered.

It is increasingly recognized that diabetic neuropathy is associated with early diabetes, prediabetes, and the metabolic syndrome. Early detection and diagnosis are important to slow progression and prevent complications. Although strict glucose control is an effective treatment in type 1 diabetes, it is less effective in type 2 diabetes. There is a growing body of literature that lifestyle interventions may be able to prevent or slow progression of neuropathy in type 2 diabetes. In addition to the typical distal symmetric polyneuropathy, there are many types of "atypical" diabetic neuropathies that are important to recognize.

Peripheral neuropathies have many nonspecific features that are shared by various neurologic disorders. These disorders include atypical peripheral neuropathies along with neurologic disorders outside of the peripheral nervous system. An understanding of clinical fundamentals and a measured approach to laboratory work-up can assist the provider in achieving diagnostic confidence.

Small fiber neuropathy is common and prevalent in the elderly. The disease can be associated with many medical conditions. It often has a negative impact on quality of life due to painful paresthesia, dizziness, and sedative side effects of pain medications. Skin biopsy is the gold standard diagnostic test. Screening for associated conditions is important, because etiology-specific treatment can slow down disease progression and ameliorate symptoms. Adequate pain control can be challenging due to safety and tolerability of pain medications in the elderly. Treatment should be individualized with the goals of controlling underlying causes, alleviating pain, and optimizing daily function.

Patients with cancer may experience neuropathy at any stage of malignancy, ranging from symptoms that are the earliest signs of cancer to side effects of treatment. Peripheral nerves are affected most commonly in a symmetric, stocking-glove pattern. Sensory neuronopathies, plexopathies, and radiculopathies may also be seen. The most common type of neuropathy in patients with cancer is related to chemotherapy, and recently peripheral nerve complications have been described as an effect of immune checkpoint inhibitors too. Other causes include paraneoplastic syndromes, direct tumor infiltration, and radiation. Treatment focuses on addressing the underlying cancer and management of neuropathic pain.

This article provides an overview of the clinical features, diagnosis, and treatment of the major paraprotein-related peripheral neuropathies, including monoclonal gammopathy of undetermined significance, Waldenström macroglobulinemia, POEMS syndrome, multiple myeloma, transthyretin amyloidosis, and light chain amyloidosis. For each paraprotein neuropathy, the epidemiology, demographics, systemic findings, and electrophysiologic features are presented. Pharmacologic treatment of transthyretin amyloid polyneuropathy also is reviewed.

Guillain-Barré syndrome (GBS) is an acute autoimmune neuropathy that can cause motor, sensory, and autonomic symptoms. Although GBS primarily is a neuropathic disorder, multiple organ systems can be affected during the disease course, and older patients may be more vulnerable to systemic complications. Close clinical monitoring and early interventions using pharmacologic and nonpharmacological treatments may lead to an improved long-term outcome.

This article discusses the chronic immune-mediated polyneuropathies, a broad category of acquired polyneuropathies that encompasses chronic inflammatory demyelinating polyradiculoneuropathy (CIDP), the most common immune-mediated neuropathy, the CIDP variants, and the vasculitic neuropathies. Polyneuropathies associated with rheumatological diseases and systemic inflammatory diseases, such as sarcoidosis, will also be briefly covered. These patients' history, examination, serum studies, and electrodiagnostic studies, as well as histopathological findings in the case of vasculitis, confirm the diagnosis and differentiate them from the more common length-dependent polyneuropathies. Prompt identification and initiation of treatment is imperative for these chronic immune-mediated polyneuropathies to prevent disability and even death.

Inflammatory peripheral neuropathies can be disabling for any patient. Selecting the most appropriate agent for treatment, especially in the elderly, is no simple task. Several factors should be considered. Herein, we discuss immunotherapeutic options for peripheral nerve diseases and the important considerations required for choosing one in the geriatric population.

Neuropathic pain is common in the geriatric population. Diagnosis requires a thorough history and physical examination to differentiate it from other types of pain. Once diagnosed, further workup is required to elucidate the cause, including potential reversible causes of neuropathy. When treating neuropathic pain in the elderly, it is important to consider patients' comorbidities and other medications to avoid drug-drug interactions and iatrogenic effects given the physiologic changes of drug metabolism in the elderly. Nonsystemic therapies and topical medications should be considered. Systemic medications should be started at low dose and titrated up slowly with frequent monitoring for adverse effects.

CLINICS IN GERIATRIC MEDICINE

SERIES OF RELATED INTEREST

Medical Clinics of North America
Primary Care: Clinics in Office Practice

THE CLINICS ARE AVAILABLE ONLINE!
Access your subscription at:
www.theclinics.com

Preface

Peripheral Neuropathy: More than Numb Feet

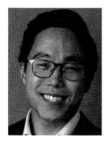

Peter H. Jin, MD
Editor

Diseases of the peripheral nerve are among the most common neurologic disorders in the geriatric population. The chief complaints of numbness, tingling, and pain in the hands and feet are commonplace in any primary care physician's practice, and "peripheral neuropathy" is a frequent diagnosis. "Peripheral neuropathy," however, is a large umbrella category with many distinct diseases. These diseases include the very common disorders of diabetic sensory polyneuropathy and carpal tunnel syndrome but also rarer diseases of autoimmune and vasculitic neuropathies. While many of these diseases have similar symptoms, the differences in expected disease course and management vary dramatically. Some diseases, such as Guillain-Barre syndrome, even require urgent or emergent medical attention to prevent mortality and disability. To further complicate matters, peripheral neuropathy is a flagship example of neurologic disease due to systemic diseases. These diseases include endocrinopathies, nutritional deficiencies, cancers, and rheumatologic disorders. Diseases of the peripheral nerve are often among the most debilitating aspects of these systemic diseases. Furthermore, peripheral neuropathy can be a heralding sign that precedes other more typical clinical findings.

There is a multitude of pathologic conditions and causes of peripheral nerve diseases, which can make evaluation and management of this condition challenging. Where do you start? When is it serious? When is it something else entirely? What treatment should you use? Good-quality care requires a keen understanding of the nuanced differences between different diseases of the peripheral nerve. Familiarity with the utility and limitations of tests, such as nerve conduction and electromyography, imaging, and biopsy, is invaluable in steering diagnostic workup. A comprehensive grasp of the various treatment options can help personalize care for patients with neuropathy. A healthy dose of humility also helps, as many of these diseases often appear clinically identical.

Clin Geriatr Med 37 (2021) xiii–xiv
https://doi.org/10.1016/j.cger.2021.02.001
0749-0690/21/© 2021 Published by Elsevier Inc.

In this series of articles, the authors provide the reader with foundational knowledge on how to approach patients with suspected peripheral neuropathy, a broad overview of the many types of peripheral neuropathy, and an overview of different treatment modalities used for symptom management and disease modification. We hope that you come away with a greater appreciation for the many diseases that often are lumped into the category of "peripheral neuropathy" and that you gain an understanding of peripheral neuropathy beyond simply the presence of numb feet.

Peter H. Jin, MD
University of Maryland School of Medicine
Department of Neurology
110 S Paca Street
Baltimore, MD 21201, USA

E-mail address:
pjin@som.umaryland.edu

A Clinical Approach to Disease of Peripheral Nerve

Rajeev Motiwala, MD

KEYWORDS

- Pattern of neuropathy • Symptoms of peripheral neuropathy
- Clinical examination in patients with suspected neuropathy • Screening • Referral

KEY POINTS

- Understand patterns of neuropathy and how they influence clinical evaluation.
- Review screening measures for neuropathy.
- Emphasize important features of history in patients with possible neuropathy.
- Learn about critical examination elements while approaching patients with suspected neuropathy.
- Recognize situations when urgent evaluation or specialty referral would be appropriate.

 Video content accompanies this article at http://www.geriatric.theclinics.com.

INTRODUCTION

Peripheral neuropathy is one of the most common neurologic problems encountered by primary care physicians and geriatricians in particular. The prevalence in general population is about 2.4%, and it increases with age to approximately 8% in those older than 55 years.[1,2]

These are conditions affecting peripheral nerves resulting in a variety of symptoms and signs, including pain, paresthesia (subjective complaint of tingling, numbness, crawling), impaired sensation, weakness, and alteration in gait.

It is important to remember that these symptoms can also result from involvement of other anatomic sites of the nervous system.

- Sensory symptoms can be caused by neuropathy, plexopathy, radiculopathy, myelopathy, and diseases involving central sensory pathways.
- Motor weakness can be caused by myopathy, neuromuscular junction disorder, neuropathy, plexopathy, radiculopathy, and diseases affecting anterior horn cells and motor pathways in the spinal cord or more central regions.

Department of Neurology, NYU Grossman School of Medicine, 222 East 41st Street, 9th Floor, New York, NY 10017, USA
E-mail address: rajeev.motiwala@nyulangone.org

Clin Geriatr Med 37 (2021) 197–208
https://doi.org/10.1016/j.cger.2021.01.009
0749-0690/21/© 2021 Elsevier Inc. All rights reserved.
geriatric.theclinics.com

A comprehensive history and physical examination often provide clues that the presenting problem is likely to be related to neuropathy.

Physicians dealing with geriatric population are faced with the following challenges:

1. When to suspect neuropathy based on symptoms
2. Routinely screen asymptomatic patients who have conditions such as diabetes mellitus, which put them at higher risk, and how to screen these patients quickly
3. How to counsel and treat patients with neuropathy
4. When to refer patients for subspecialty evaluation

PATTERN OF NEUROPATHY

The clinical presentation will vary depending on the pattern of neuropathy. Length-dependent neuropathies involve the longest nerve fibers first and tend to affect distal lower extremities at the onset. Non–length-dependent neuropathies can involve fibers regardless of length, and the symptoms can involve proximal and distal body parts, trunk, and face. If large fibers are involved predominantly, weakness and ataxia can result. Involvement of small fibers will cause pain and allodynia (pain elicited by non-noxious stimuli) without significant weakness. The most common pattern of neuropathy is characterized by length-dependent involvement of predominantly sensory fibers, both small and large. One or more large peripheral nerves can be involved, leading to asymmetric weakness and sensory loss as seen in mononeuritis simplex or multiplex. Autonomic fibers can be affected in addition to other nerve fibers, or they can be affected predominantly in isolation, resulting in specific features such as orthostatic hypotension, abnormalities of sweating, abnormalities of sphincter function, and sexual function.

It may be useful to conceptualize neuropathy based on anatomic pattern (**Fig. 1**) and size of nerve fibers involved (**Fig. 2**), and this will account for variability in symptoms and signs between different patients.[3,4]

Historical elements that are important to address in a patient with suspected neuropathy:

1. Onset and time course:[3–5]
   - Acute onset and rapid progression may be seen in conditions such as Guillain-Barré syndrome, toxicity of chemotherapy, critical illness, vasculitis, infections.

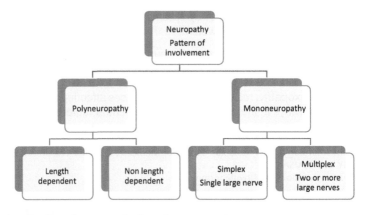

Fig. 1. Classification of neuropathy based on anatomic pattern.

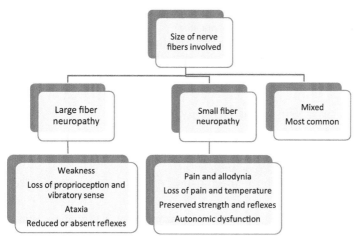

Fig. 2. Classification of neuropathy based on size of nerve fibers involved.

- Subacute onset and progression can be seen in chronic inflammatory demyelinating neuropathy, paraneoplastic neuropathy, and nutritional deficiency states.
- Chronic or insidious onset with slow progression is the most common presentation in an outpatient setting. Causative conditions include diabetes, chronic alcohol use, and hereditary neuropathy (often unsuspected).

2. Associated comorbidities often provide a clue to the possible cause of neuropathy, and many of these conditions can be uncovered by comprehensive medical history:
   - Diabetes mellitus
   - History of chronic alcohol use
   - Other metabolic conditions such as thyroid disease and renal failure
   - Recent change in diet, weight loss, gastrointestinal disorders, and bariatric surgery leading to vitamin deficiencies, particularly vitamin B12 (cyanocobalamin) and vitamin B1 (thiamine)
   - History of underlying malignancy or treatment with chemotherapeutic agents
   - Human immunodeficiency virus (HIV) infection
   - Skin rash, arthritis, and known rheumatologic or autoimmune disease
   - History of possible environmental or occupational exposure (heavy metals, pesticides)

3. Many medications can cause or contribute to development of neuropathy. Some notable common offending agents include the following:[6]
   - Antimicrobials: fluoroquinolones, metronidazole, nitrofurantoin, isoniazid, ethambutol, linezolid
   - Chemotherapeutic agents: vincristine, docetaxel, paclitaxel, oxaliplatin, thalidomide, bortezomib
   - Cardiovascular agent: amiodarone
   - Pyridoxine (vitamin B6): high doses often self-administered from health food sources
   - Nucleoside reverse-transcriptase inhibitors (antiretroviral agents) used for treatment of HIV infection: zalcitabine, didanosine, stavudine, lamivudine (newer agents are less likely to be responsible)
   - Statins: the association is not strong for clinically significant neuropathy but well described

- Immunosuppressants: biologics, interferons, leflunomide
- Others: phenytoin, levodopa, disulfiram
4. Family history of neuropathy: patients with hereditary neuropathy would be expected to present at a younger age. However, it is not rare for patients to present later in life, particularly with milder forms of neuropathy. It is thought that some of the previously undiagnosed or cryptogenic cases may belong to this group.

SYMPTOMS OF PERIPHERAL NEUROPATHY

A typical patient with neuropathy is likely to report tingling and numbness in feet, recurrent episodes of sharp pain in toes, and mild lack of balance. The symptoms tend to evolve as the condition progresses.

The symptoms of peripheral neuropathy can be broadly conceptualized in many ways:

1. Symptoms related to involvement of sensory fibers, motor fibers, and autonomic fibers
2. Symptoms caused by involvement of small nerve fibers and large nerve fibers
3. Positive and negative symptoms depending on presumed mechanism of uninhibited activity or reduced activity of nerve fibers

Different symptoms of neuropathy can be attributed to involvement of sensory fibers, motor fibers, and autonomic fibers within the peripheral nerves (**Table 1**). Trophic changes are believed to be related to a variety of factors, including loss of neurotrophic factors. Many neuropathies result in dysfunction of all types of fibers, but some conditions can result in greater involvement of one subset over others.

Positive symptoms may result from uninhibited or abnormal spontaneous nerve activity, and these may include pain, cramps, and twitching. The type of pain can be quite variable. Neuropathic pain is described as burning, sharp, electric shock-like, but it can also be reported as deep aching pain. It is often useful to ask the patients to localize the pain whether it is on the surface or deep seated. In most length-dependent neuropathies the patients may initially complain that their feet feel as if

Table 1 Symptoms of neuropathy	
Sensory	Numbness or loss of sensation
	Pain, tingling, burning feet
	Allodynia: pain elicited by a stimulus that generally should not induce pain
	Hyperalgesia: pain response is exaggerated after a stimulus that is capable of eliciting pain
	Paresthesia: tingling, crawling sensation described by the patient
	Unsteady gait and falls
Motor	Weakness: difficulty gripping objects, tendency to trip easily
	Loss of muscle mass
	Muscle twitching
	Muscle cramps
Autonomic	Postural dizziness and syncope
	Sexual dysfunction: erectile dysfunction, retrograde ejaculation
	Bladder involvement
	Easy satiety, constipation, or diarrhea
	Dryness of mouth, eyes, and skin
Trophic	Skin and joint changes
	Skin discoloration, callus, skin ulcers, enlarged joints (Charcot joints)

they are wrapped in stockings. The pain of neuropathy is often more noticeable at rest and during night.

Negative symptoms reflect reduced nerve activity and result in loss of sensation, weakness, ataxia, and atrophy. Patients with distal sensory loss may complain about delayed wound healing and tendency to lose balance after closing eyes or in dark surroundings.

The patients with distal weakness may develop hammer toes and complain of reduced grip strength. When the weakness spreads more proximally, they may report difficulty getting out of low chairs and problems climbing stairs. Recurrent tripping while stepping off curbs may reflect partial foot drop. More chronic conditions can result in deformities such as pes cavus.

Patients with mononeuropathy such as median neuropathy at wrist or carpal tunnel syndrome will complain about pain and nocturnal paresthesia in the affected hand. The symptoms of ulnar neuropathy may include tingling along the inner aspect of forearm and fourth and fifth fingers with numbness of those fingers. These symptoms may be triggered by elbow movements. A patient with radial nerve palsy may wake up with a wrist drop. Peroneal or fibular neuropathy can result in a foot drop but the patient may report slapping gait or tendency for the ankle to "turn" easily.

CLINICAL EXAMINATION IN PATIENTS WITH SUSPECTED NEUROPATHY

This is likely to vary depending on whether the intention is to screen patients for neuropathy who have known conditions such as diabetes mellitus or to evaluate patients presenting with clinical symptoms suggesting peripheral neuropathy.

Screening can be performed by using 2 or more tests:[7]

- Light touch perception using 10-g Semmes-Weinstein monofilament examination (cotton swab or cotton wisp is often substituted in clinical practice)
- Superficial pain or pinprick perception using a sharp pin or sharp end of a wooden stick
- Vibration testing with a 128 Hz tuning fork.
- Testing of ankle deep tendon reflexes

Annual screening is important in patients with known diabetes. Clanging tuning fork test may be used to replace the 10-g monofilament test as the recommended technique for detection of diabetic polyneuropathy.[8] It is important to remember age-related decline in vibration sense and ankle reflexes in patients older than 65 years.[9,10] These findings in otherwise healthy elderly people can obscure distinction from polyneuropathy.[11] An elderly individual with no symptoms and no risk factors for neuropathy is unlikely to have polyneuropathy simply based on the findings of decreased distal vibratory sensation and depressed or absent ankle reflexes. Positive findings on these screening tests should prompt further diagnostic workup.

The physical examination can help confirm the diagnosis of neuropathy suspected based on history and also provide more detailed information on what nerve fiber types may be affected (**Table 2**). Most nonneurologists do not feel comfortable performing a formal neurologic examination, but focusing on various test maneuvers that allow assessment of different components of the peripheral nerves may be useful. The examination also helps rule out other causes of weakness or sensory loss such as myopathy, radiculopathy, and central disorders. Presence of spasticity and hyperreflexia as seen in patients with upper motor neuron disorders would direct the examiner away from peripheral neuropathy as being the principal diagnosis.

1. Motor examination

Table 2
Summary of physical findings depending on type of nerve fibers involved

Type of Peripheral Nerve Fibers Involved	Signs
Sensory	Glove and stocking sensory loss Sensory ataxia Positive Romberg sign Reduced or absent reflexes Pseudoathetosis
Motor	Distal weakness Atrophy and fasciculations in some cases Reduced or absent reflexes
Autonomic	Orthostatic hypotension Skin changes Abnormal sweating patterns Hyperemia or pallor
Trophic	Callus Painless ulcers in neuropathic joints Skin thinning and color changes Loss of hair in distal legs Nail changes

2. Sensory examination
3. Reflexes
4. Gait, Romberg sign
5. Assessment of autonomic dysfunction
6. Relevant cerebellar and cranial nerve examination
7. General examination

MOTOR EXAMINATION
Inspection

The classic teaching is that motor examination starts with inspection. In chronic neuropathies, one may expect to find signs of muscle atrophy in distal muscles. The small muscles of feet may develop atrophy, and there may be prominence of intermetatarsal spaces in feet, loss of prominence of extensor digitorum brevis muscle bulk over lateral aspect of dorsum of foot, and loss of plantar muscle fullness. In the upper extremities, there may be loss of muscle mass in the first web space over the dorsal aspect of hand and flattening of thenar and hypothenar muscle prominences. Intermittent spontaneous muscle twitching or fasciculations can be seen in some patients with neuropathy, although this finding is more prominent in anterior horn cell disorders.

Tone

The muscle tone is evaluated most commonly by moving different joints passively and judging resistance to passive range of motion. There will be reduced resistance and "floppiness" when tone is reduced in the presence of significant neuropathy.

Strength

It is useful to determine if the muscle weakness is symmetrical or asymmetrical. If it is asymmetrical, does it correspond to a single large nerve distribution? In length-dependent neuropathies, the weakness first involves distal muscles of lower extremities. Proximal muscle involvement in addition to distal muscle weakness in early stages can be seen with inflammatory neuropathies such as acute inflammatory demyelinating polyneuropathy and chronic inflammatory demyelinating polyneuropathy.

There are limitations to confrontational strength testing. The muscle strength often depends on patient's age, overall body habitus, conditioning, presence or absence of pain, and relative strength compared with the examiner. Incorporating functional testing may reveal specific functional disabilities along with subtle weakness that is often missed on confrontational strength testing. The patient may be asked to stand up from a seated position without support of the chair or perform knee bends to assess the proximal lower extremity strength. Walking on heels can allow detection of mild ankle dorsiflexor muscle weakness. Walking on toes can detect subtle ankle plantar flexor muscle weakness.

SENSORY EXAMINATION

Sensory symptoms and sensory findings often precede motor weakness in most common neuropathies. The sensory examination in its full extent involves testing of primary sensory modalities of light touch, pain, temperature, vibration, and proprioception (joint position). Testing of cortical sensory modalities includes evaluation of graphesthesia, stereognosis, and presence of sensory hemineglect. A detailed examination can become fairly tedious, and patient cooperation is paramount. A tailored approach based on patient's symptoms and the purpose of examination (screening or diagnostic) can guide the practitioner. In a patient with no sensory complaints, testing with a cotton wisp, pin, and tuning fork in feet may suffice.

It is important to remember that "large fibers" convey sensation of fine light touch, vibration, and proprioception (joint movement). These sensory modalities are tested with the help of a cotton wisp, tuning fork, and passive joint movements. "Small fibers" typically carry impulses from receptors responsible for perception of crude touch, pain, and temperature. These sensations are tested by response to sensation of cold and pin prick.

In most peripheral neuropathies, the sensory findings are prominent distally in lower extremities and then spread proximally as the condition progresses. Fingers can be involved after the symptoms have spread up to knees or lower thighs. It is useful to start sensory examination distally and compare distal segments with proximal segments, one side with the other side, and lower extremities with upper extremities. The classic pattern of sensory loss in peripheral neuropathy is "glove and stocking" type. It is important to remember that the sensation may not be absent and may simply show relative reduction in intensity and "distal to proximal gradient." It is unusual to find a sensory level on the trunk with loss of sensation below that level—this finding should raise consideration for an alternative localization such as spinal cord disease.

Light touch can be tested by using a cotton wisp or cotton swab starting distally and comparing distal segment with proximal and one side with the other. Sensation of pain is also assessed in a similar fashion using the sharp end of a stick, a safety pin, or a medipin. These are discarded after single use. Sensory examination over trunk can be reserved for patients who report sensory symptoms in that area or if the sensory loss in lower extremities extends up to the groin. Patients with diabetic truncal neuropathy may have sensory loss over contiguous thoracic dermatomes. Sensation of cold is often assessed by applying the cool metallic surface of tuning fork to skin. The tuning fork can be run under cold water first to enhance sensitivity.

Vibration sense is best tested using a 128-Hz frequency tuning fork. The examiner should lightly tap the end of the tuning fork and place it against bony prominences, inner part of first metatarsophalangeal joint, or medial malleolus in the lower extremity and knuckles in the upper extremity. The examiner can serve as control, and if the patient reports not feeling vibration at all or reports that it stops before the examiner stops feeling it, some degree of vibratory loss is confirmed. If the vibration sense is absent distally, more proximal bony prominences should be assessed until a relatively normal sensation is detected. In one study, the mean duration of vibration sensation was 10.2 seconds and results of monofilament testing were abnormal only in those patients whose vibration perception was less than or equal to 4 seconds. The same study showed that "clanging tuning fork" test can detect diabetic peripheral neuropathy earlier and more accurately than 10-g monofilament test, and it should be used as the recommended technique for detection of diabetic peripheral neuropathy.[8]

Joint position sense is tested by moving interphalangeal joints of fingers and toes through a small range of movement while supporting the base of the digit proximally. If the joint position is absent in distal joints, more proximal joints should be tested. Patients who have significant proprioceptive loss may show presence of abnormal movements in the fingers of outstretched hands when their eyes are closed—this is called pseudoathetosis.[12]

Sensory loss in a pattern that differs from the typical distal or length-dependent pattern should prompt consideration of other diagnoses. If the sensory loss is in a dermatomal pattern, one may suspect radiculopathy. If the sensory loss conforms to a large peripheral nerve, a diagnosis of mononeuropathy should be entertained. For example, sensory loss along the lateral aspect of forearm and thumb would suggest C6 radiculopathy, and sensory loss over lateral aspect of leg and dorsum of foot may be consistent with peroneal neuropathy or L5 radiculopathy.

REFLEXES

The deep tendon reflexes are normal in patients with small fiber neuropathy. They are diminished or absent in patients with large fiber neuropathy, as an intact reflex arc is essential. The reflex arc includes sensory fibers, synapse within the spinal segment, and motor pathway. The reflexes will first be affected distally in a length-dependent fashion. The ankle reflexes will be diminished or absent. A significant asymmetry of reflexes is unusual and should suggest other associated condition. The patients in this age group may have coexisting radiculopathy, which would cause asymmetrical loss of reflexes or a condition such as cervical spondylotic myelopathy that may lead to relative preservation or prominence of deep tendon reflexes even in the face of neuropathy.

GAIT

Examination of gait can assess several neurologic functions. It is possible to judge balance by observing tandem gait, proximal lower extremity strength as indicated by stability of pelvis and hip musculature, and distal lower extremity strength as demonstrated by ability to walk on heels and toes. The patients may report their subjective experience by describing that when they walk barefoot there is a sensation of walking on cracked glass or as if they are walking on cotton wool. The patients sometimes refer to unsteadiness as dizziness, and it is important to encourage them to explain in more detail what they are actually experiencing.

Abnormal gait is an important cause of frequent falls in the elderly.[13,14] There are several mechanical and neurologic causes of abnormal gait, and peripheral neuropathy is an important cause. There are different gait patterns depending on the predominant deficit, proprioceptive loss, motor weakness, or presence of pain (**Table 3**).

Romberg sign is a test of proprioception, but it is often assessed during gait examination. Before the patient is asked to walk, it is useful to have them stand with feet close together after assuring a steady base. The patient is then asked to close their eyes, and the examiner stands close by to provide support if necessary. The patient may sway or lose balance and fall if Romberg sign is positive. This finding suggests proprioceptive loss, and when visual compensation is removed, the deficit becomes obvious. If the patient cannot stand with feet close together with eyes open, as in case of cerebellar disorders, Romberg test cannot be performed.

AUTONOMIC FUNCTION

A detailed assessment of autonomic function is outside the scope of a routine office examination. Some of the simple tests include checking for presence of orthostatic hypotension, abnormal sweating pattern, and changes in skin color or temperature. A drop in systolic blood pressure greater than 20 mm Hg and or diastolic blood pressure greater than 10 mm Hg in 3 minutes after assuming an upright position indicates orthostatic hypotension.[15] In patients with autonomic neuropathy (they may have evidence of more generalized neuropathy in addition), there may be lack of compensatory tachycardia.

OTHER NEUROLOGIC EXAMINATION

Patients with neuropathy can have abnormalities in other aspects of the neurologic examination also. Patients with Guillain-Barré syndrome often have bilateral facial weakness. Diabetic neuropathy may be associated with pupillary abnormalities. Cerebellar examination is important to distinguish sensory ataxia from cerebellar ataxia. Dysarthria and nystagmus can be seen with cerebellar disorders and not with neuropathy.

Table 3
Abnormal gait patterns in neuropathy

Type of Gait	Description	Cause
Ataxic	Unsteady, wide based	Large fiber or proprioceptive loss
Stomping	The foot is raised higher than normal, and it is brought down harder	Often a component of ataxic gait due to loss of proprioception
Steppage gait	The ankle hangs with toes pointing down, the leg has to be lifted higher for toes to clear the ground	Weakness of ankle dorsiflexion
Antalgic gait	Cautious, slow, often unable to walk barefoot due to pain in soles	Small fiber involvement with hyperalgesia of soles

GENERAL EXAMINATION

A thorough general examination may reveal abnormalities in patients with neuropathy. Some examples are presence of orthostatic hypotension, suggesting autonomic involvement, glossitis in vitamin B12 deficiency, skeletal deformities such as pes cavus and scoliosis in hereditary neuropathy, skin rash in patients with vasculitis, and connective tissue disorders.

RECOMMENDED "BARE MINIMUM" EXAMINATION IN PATIENTS WITH SUSPECTED NEUROPATHY

As demonstrated in Video 1,

- Check at least one proximal muscle group in upper extremities by asking them to raise both arms fully against gravity and resistance.
- Check distal muscles in upper extremity by confirming that the hand grip is strong and symmetric on both sides.
- Check gait. Is the gait steady and narrow based? Can the patient stand up without assistance and walk on heels, toes, and perform tandem gait? This will also allow assessment of proximal and distal lower extremity muscle strength.
- Check sensation in feet; vibration and pin prick.
- Check ankle reflexes.

HOW CAN INITIAL EVALUATION POINT TOWARD POSSIBLE CAUSE OF NEUROPATHY IN PATIENTS?

Further workup of neuropathy will be addressed in subsequent chapters. It is clear that a shotgun approach to diagnosis with a large number of blood tests and electrodiagnostic studies is not cost-effective in most patients with neuropathy. The initial clinical evaluation, assessment of risk factors, and recognizing specific patterns of neuropathy can be of tremendous help.

- An acute or subacute onset suggests immune-mediated or infectious process.
- A chronic or insidious onset indicates metabolic, toxic, or hereditary cause.
- Diabetes mellitus is possibly the most common cause of neuropathy in geriatric population. Neuropathic symptoms may be seen in patients with impaired glucose tolerance before development of overt diabetes.[16,17]
- A comprehensive evaluation that includes medical history, neurologic examination, simple screening laboratory tests, and electrodiagnostic studies yields an etiologic diagnosis in 74% to 82% of patients with polyneuropathy.[18]
- Small fiber neuropathy can be idiopathic but it is also common in diabetic patients.
- Prominent autonomic component suggests diabetes, amyloidosis, and autoimmune causes.

PATIENTS WITH SUSPECTED NEUROPATHY WHO SHOULD BE CONSIDERED FOR NEUROLOGIC CONSULTATION AND ADDITIONAL DIAGNOSTIC STUDIES

- Acute onset
- Rapidly progressive
- Severe functional limitation
- Significant asymmetry
- Pure or predominant motor symptoms
- Pure or predominant autonomic symptoms

- Bulbar symptoms including difficulties in speech, swallowing, and breathing
- Mononeuropathy multiplex

TREATMENT

The various aspects of specific treatment depending on the cause of neuropathy will be addressed in subsequent chapters. The treatment rationale is guided by the following principles:

- It is critical to identify those patients who need specialty referral, urgent intervention, or hospitalization, for example, patients with Guillain-Barré syndrome.
- Specific treatment measures include optimizing blood glucose control in patients with diabetes, reducing or removing exposure to offending agents such as alcohol, correction of vitamin deficiency, and addressing metabolic factors such as hypothyroidism.
- Demyelinating neuropathies in particular may be amenable to immunomodulatory therapies.
- Symptomatic treatment includes use of various agents to control neuropathic pain.
- Proper foot care, fall prevention, physical therapy, occupational therapy, use of orthotics, and other assistive devices for ambulation are often the most important long-term and ongoing interventions that can improve the quality of life.

CLINICS CARE POINTS

- The prevalence in general population is about 2.4%, and it increases with age to approximately 8% in those older than 55 years.
- Neuropathies can be length dependent with distal predominance, non–length dependent or can involve individual large nerves as in mononeuropathy simplex and mononeuropathy multiplex.
- Clinical symptoms and physical findings vary depending on whether small nerve fibers, large nerve fibers, or both types of nerve fibers are involved.
- Screening for presence of neuropathy can be accomplished quickly by testing feet with light touch, pin prick, or 128-Hz tuning fork and by checking ankle reflexes. Testing of vibratory sense is the most single reliable test.
- The onset, time course, associated medical conditions, medications, and family history are important historical elements.
- A comprehensive examination in patients suspected to have neuropathy includes motor examination, sensory examination, reflexes, and gait assessment in addition to pertinent elements of rest of the nervous system and general physical examination.
- It is important to recognize conditions that may potentially progress rapidly or require specific therapeutic intervention.

ACKNOWLEDGMENTS

Arielle Kurzweil, MD, Associate Professor of Neurology, NYU Grossman School of Medicine. Hao Huang, MD, Fellow, Headache Medicine, Department of Neurology, NYU Grossman School of Medicine.

DISCLOSURE

The author has no disclosures.

SUPPLEMENTARY DATA

Supplementary data related to this article can be found online at https://doi.org/10.1016/j.cger.2021.01.009.

REFERENCES

1. Martyn CN, Hughes RAC. Epidemiology of peripheral neuropathy. J Neurol Neurosurg Psychiatry 1997;62(4):310–8.
2. Italian General Practitioner Study Group (IGPSG). Chronic symmetric symptomatic polyneuropathy in elderly: a field screening investigation in two Italian regions, I: prevalence and general characteristics of the sample. Neurology 1995;45(10):1832–6.
3. Hughes RAC. Peripheral neuropathy. BMJ 2002;324:466–9.
4. England JD, Asbury AK. Peripheral neuropathy. Lancet 2004;363:2151–61.
5. Watson JC, Dyck PJB. Peripheral neuropathy: a practical approach to diagnosis and symptom management. Mayo Clinic Proc 2015;90(7):940–51.
6. Jones MR, Urits I, Wolf J, et al. Drug-induced peripheral neuropathy: a narrative review. Curr Clin Pharmacol 2020;l 5:38–48.
7. Perkins BA, Olaleye D, Zinman B, et al. Simple screening tests for peripheral neuropathy in diabetes clinic. Diabetes Care 2001;242(2):250–6.
8. Oyer D, Saxon D, Shah A. Quantitative assessment of diabetic peripheral neuropathy with use of the clanging tuning fork test. Endocr Pract 2007;13(1):5–10.
9. Odenheimer G, Funkenstein HH, Beckett L, et al. Comparison of neurologic changes in 'successfully aging' persons vs the total aging population. Arch Neurol 1994 Jun;5 l(6):573–80.
10. Gladstone DJ, Black SE. The neurological examination in aging, dementia and cerebrovascular disease. Geriatrics and Aging. 2002;5(7):36–43.
11. Vrancken AF, Kalmijn S, Brugman F, et al. The meaning of distal sensory loss and absent ankle reflexes in relation to age. A meta-analysis. J Neurol 2006;253:578–89.
12. Lo YL. See S. Pseudoathetosis. N Engl J Med 2010;363(19):e29.
13. Verghese J, Ambrose AF, Lipton RB, et al. Neurological gait abnormalities and risk of falls in older adults. J Neuro 2010;257(3):392–8.
14. Pirker W, Katzenschlager R. Gait disorders in adults and the elderly. Wien Klin Wochenschr 2017;129(3):81–95.
15. Lanier JB, Mote MB, Clay EC. Evaluation and management of orthostatic hypotension. Am Fam Physician 2011;84(5):527–36.
16. Singleton JR, Smith AG, Broomberg MB. Increased prevalence of impaired glucose tolerance in patients with painful sensory neuropathy. Diabetes care 2001;24(8):1448–53.
17. Singleton JR, Smith AG, Broomberg MB. Painful sensory polyneuropathy associated with impaired glucose tolerance. Muscle Nerve 2001;24(9):1225–8.
18. England JD, Gronseth GS, Franklin G, et al. Practice Parameter: evaluation of distal symmetric polyneuropathy: role of laboratory and genetic testing (an evidence based review): report of the American Academy of Neurology, American association of neuromuscular and electrodiagnostic medicine, and American Academy of Physical Medicine and Rehabilitation. Neurology 2009;72(2):185–92.

Electrodiagnostic Testing for Disorders of Peripheral Nerves

Joseph M. Choi, MD[a,b,*], Gianluca Di Maria, MD[c]

KEYWORDS

- Polyneuropathy • Nerve conduction studies • Electromyography • CTS
- Ulnar neuropathy • Radiculopathy

KEY POINTS

- Diagnosis of peripheral nerve disease can be clinically challenging, and electrodiagnostic study (EDX) is a valuable diagnostic tool to confirm diagnosis of polyneuropathy, compressive mononeuropathy, and radiculopathy.
- Nerve conduction studies have high sensitivity and specificity for compressive neuropathies.
- Needle electromyography has moderate sensitivity but very high specificity for diagnosing cervical and lumbosacral radiculopathy.
- The EDX study design is based on the referral question. The EDX referral form that has a clinical diagnosis (eg, left carpal tunnel syndrome) or symptom (right foot drop) will allow proper study design to achieve higher yield.
- Electrophysiological findings are best applied in the clinical context to correctly diagnose neuromuscular disease.

INTRODUCTION

Prevalence of neuropathies is 2% to 3% in the general population, but this increases to 8% when patients are older than 55 years.[1] Electrodiagnostic studies, such as nerve conduction studies (NCS) and electromyography (EMG), provide a tool for localization of disease and assessment of its disease severity. NCS are helpful in diagnosing various neuropathies, and needle EMG is more helpful with radiculopathies

[a] Georgetown University, Washington, DC, USA; [b] Department of Neurology, MedStar Washington Hospital Center, MedStar Georgetown University Hospital, 3800 Reservoir Road, PHC 7th Floor, Washington, DC 20007, USA; [c] Department of Neurology, MedStar Georgetown University Hospital, 3800 Reservoir Road, PHC 7th Floor, Washington, DC 20007, USA
* Corresponding author. Department of Neurology, MedStar Washington Hospital Center, MedStar Georgetown University Hospital, 3800 Reservoir Road, PHC 7th Floor, Washington, DC 20007.
E-mail address: joseph.m.choi@gunet.georgetown.edu

Clin Geriatr Med 37 (2021) 209–221
https://doi.org/10.1016/j.cger.2021.01.010
0749-0690/21/© 2021 Elsevier Inc. All rights reserved.

and myopathies.[2–6] NCS and needle EMG are separate tests but are used in combination during routine neurophysiological testing.

As with all diagnostic studies, the results should be interpreted with the clinical history and examination in mind. An electrophysiological diagnosis does not necessarily give cause of the disease. For example, an EDX conclusion of axonal sensory polyneuropathy cannot distinguish if the polyneuropathy is due to diabetes or from B12 deficiency. The referring clinician needs to put the finding into clinical context.

EDX is a 2-part evaluation, and it is beneficial to explain to the patient what will happen during this study. The first part is the NCS and involves a patient receiving electrical impulses in their hand or hands or leg or legs. The electrical stimulations are very brief, and there are no residual side effects. Implanted cardiac pacemaker/defibrillator or left ventricular assist devices are not contraindicated.[7]

The second part of the test is the needle EMG. A small, sterile EMG needle will be inserted in the muscles. This insertion usually causes some transient pain and discomfort while the needle is in the muscle. There is a possibility of small bruising, but this can be reduced by applying pressure at the site. Patients can be on antiplatelet agents during the test, but higher risk exists for patients on anticoagulants.[6–8] If the patient is on an anticoagulant for a limited time, then it is generally advisable to wait until they have discontinued the anticoagulant before testing. If clinically necessary, the needle EMG can be conducted while on anticoagulants, but fewer muscles will be tested to reduce the chance of hematoma and other complications.[6–8] The test usually takes 30 to 60 minutes, and there is no activity restriction posttest.

Basics of Nerve Conduction Study and Electromyography

Diseases of the peripheral nervous system can affect muscles (myopathies), nerves (neuropathies), and neuromuscular junctions (myasthenia gravis), sometimes in combination. Peripheral neuropathies can impair sensory, motor, or autonomic function, either alone or in combination. They can affect the cell body (eg, neuronopathy or ganglionopathy), the myelin, and the axon (axonopathy). EDX allows the study of the sensory neuron, motor neuron, neuromuscular junction, and muscle individually by using a combination of NCS and needle EMG. Used together, they are a valuable diagnostic aid for neuromuscular disease.

Nerve conduction studies

NCS are used to assess peripheral nerves. There are 3 main types of peripheral nerves: sensory, motor, and autonomic nerves. On NCS, only large-fiber sensory and motor neurons are assessed. Motor nerve study is separate from sensory nerve study, so which type of nerves are affected can be differentiated. In addition to assessing different nerve types, the NCS can tell you what part of the nerve is affected, myelin versus axons.

In motor NCS, an electrical stimulus is applied on the surface of the skin above a given nerve, and an action potential of motor nerves (compound muscle action potential, CMAP) over a belly of a muscle is recorded. In sensory NCS, an electrical stimulation is applied on the surface of the skin and the response (sensory nerve action potential, SNAP) is recorded on the skin over a distal segment of the nerve.[9] This action potential represents the number of fibers that depolarize after an external electrical stimulus is applied. Three major features are observed and measured: Amplitude, distal latency, and conduction velocity (**Fig. 1**). By these 3 features, it can be distinguished whether the neuropathy is due to problems in the myelin sheath or the axons (**Table 1**).

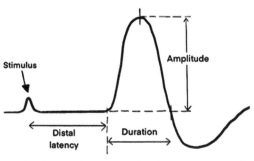

Fig. 1. Motor nerve conduction study. Three major features measured: amplitude, distal latency, and conduction velocity.

- Axonal neuropathy: Characterized by reduced amplitude of the CMAP, normal distal latency, and conduction velocity. If the axonal injury is severe, you can have preferential loss of faster nerve fibers where you can see mild slowing of nerve conduction velocity.[9] This can be reported as a mixed finding whereby there are minor demyelinating features seen on the NCS. The causes of axonal neuropathies are extensive, but some of the more common causes are *metabolic* (eg, diabetes), nutritional deficiencies (eg, B12), medications (eg, *chemotherapy*), infection (eg, HIV), and systemic disease (eg, uremia and hypothyroidism).
- *Demyelinating neuropathy*: Characterized by increased distal latency and decreased conduction velocity. Demyelinating polyneuropathy is less common than axonal neuropathy. The demyelinating disease generally has a more rapid course and usually responds to treatment. Urgent neurology evaluation is necessary. The most common acquired demyelinating polyneuropathies are Guillain-Barre syndrome (GBS) and chronic inflammatory demyelinating polyneuropathy (CIDP).

Electromyography

EMG can be very helpful in distinguishing myopathies from neuropathies, and it is essential in diagnosing radiculopathies.[1–7] In the needle EMG, the electromyographer inserts a small needle containing a recording electrode into a selected muscle. With needle EMG, you can clearly distinguish weakness caused by neuropathy or by myopathy (**Table 2**). The needle EMG is vital in localizing radiculopathy to specific myotomes.[9–13]

- Finding on radiculopathies: In radiculopathies older than 3 weeks, the needle EMG will show abnormal spontaneous activity in the form of fibrillations, positive sharp waves, and sometimes fasciculations. If the radiculopathy is older than 3 to 4 months, the motor unit action potential (MUAP) morphology will be of long-

Table 1		
Nerve conduction studies: findings in axonal versus demyelinating disease		
	Axonal Degeneration	Demyelination
Amplitude	Decreased or absent	Reduced or normal
Distal latency	Normal	Prolonged
Conduction velocity	Normal	Slowed

Table 2
Needle electromyography findings to differentiate neurogenic versus myopathic disease

EMG Findings	Spontaneous Activities		MUAP Morphology			
	Positive Sharp Waves or Fibrillation Potential	Fasciculations	Amplitude	Duration	Polyphasic	Recruitment
Neurogenic disease	Yes	Yes	Large	Long	Yes	Reduced
Myopathic disease	Yes	No	Small	Short	No	Early

duration, large-amplitude polyphasic units that show reduced recruitment. If the needle EMGs are done less than 3 weeks from onset of symptoms, you may not see any abnormalities.

- Findings on sensorimotor polyneuropathies: If the patient has mild distal sensorimotor polyneuropathy in the feet, the needle EMG can be normal. If the neuropathies are severe, the needle EMG can show abnormal spontaneous activity in the form of fibrillations and positive sharp waves. Similar to chronic radiculopathies, on longstanding chronic and severe polyneuropathies, the MUAP morphology will be of long-duration, large-amplitude polyphasic units that show reduced recruitment.
- Finding on myopathies: EMG may show abnormal spontaneous activity in the form of fibrillations and positive sharp waves. The MUAP morphology will be of short-duration and low-amplitude units that show early recruitment pattern.

Common Symptoms Where Electrodiagnostic Study Testing Will be Helpful in Clinical Practice

Numbness and tingling in the hands

Elderly patients coming in for hand pain or weakness is very common. The usual neurologic causes are median neuropathy across the wrist (carpal tunnel syndrome [CTS]) or ulnar neuropathy across the elbow or cervical radiculopathy. Electrodiagnostic testing is very helpful in differentiating these 3 diagnoses. In the elderly population, however, it is not unusual to find multiple abnormalities. The clinician must synthesize the electrodiagnostic information with the clinical findings to conclude which problem should be treated to address the patient's symptoms.

Median neuropathy across the wrist (CTS) is one of the most common reasons for referral for EDX. The study has high sensitivity and specificity for CTS, so it is a very useful test. In a compressive neuropathy like CTS, the abnormality is focal, and NCS will show slow nerve speed across the carpal tunnel space but not at other median nerve sites. The focal slowing is typically seen in both motor and sensory median nerve studies.

- Sensory NCS will reveal prolongation of distal peak latency and slowing of the conduction velocity across the wrist. **Fig. 2** shows an enlarged median sensory nerve at the carpal tunnel space, where the electrical impulse is traveling slower through that space.
- In motor NCS, there will also be prolongation of distal latency. **Fig. 3** shows an inflamed and enlarged median motor nerve at the carpal tunnel space, where

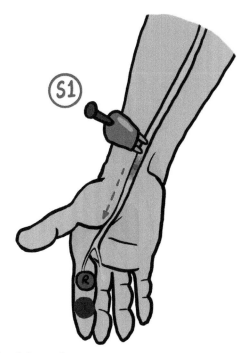

Fig. 2. Sensory study of the median nerve.

the electrical impulse is traveling slower, but speed of electrical impulse is normal at the forearm.
- In early and mild CTS, sensory nerve study may be the only part that is abnormal. As disease progresses, the motor nerve will eventually be affected.

When Should I Order Nerve Conduction Studies for Carpal Tunnel Syndrome?

If you are confident of the clinical diagnosis of CTS and the disease appears mild (episodic pain, no weakness or atrophy of thenar muscle), then it is reasonable to hold off on EDX and use conservative treatment, such as wrist splint and physical therapy. The authors recommend ordering the EDX if there is muscle atrophy or you are considering surgical evaluation. EDX will help confirm the diagnosis, assess the severity of the disease, and rule out other mimickers of CTS. You should consider performing EDX if a patient does not respond to CTS splints, if you have clinical uncertainty, or if you feel that there could be multiple causes for the patients' symptoms.

How Sensitive Is Electrodiagnostic Study in Detecting Carpal Tunnel Syndrome?

The sensitivity of NCS in detecting median neuropathy across the wrist is about 95%.[9] A small percentage of mild cases will not be diagnosed by NCS. Conservative treatment should still be initiated in patients with a normal NCS and clinical symptoms of CTS. If the symptoms worsen, repeat NCS would likely become diagnostic.

If you are suspecting CTS, it is best to put "evaluate for CTS" on the EDX referral form. An EDX test is designed for the specific disease. Correctly designing the study increases the sensitivity of the test. For example, mixed palmar nerve comparison study has high sensitivity for CTS (~95%), but this technique is not used on a routine

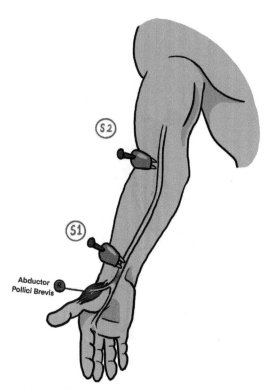

Fig. 3. Motor study of the median nerve.

screening study whereby CTS is not the referral question. If only the routine median nerve conductions are studied, the sensitivity will be lowered to about 70%.

ULNAR NEUROPATHY

Ulnar neuropathy patients primarily complain of hand weakness rather than pain. This complaint is not unusual because most of the intrinsic hand muscles are innervated by the ulnar nerve. When asked, they usually have more sensory complaints at the fourth and fifth digit, but do not be surprised if they say the sensation feels normal on all fingers.

Ulnar neuropathy: Compression at the elbow is more common than at the wrist.

- Sensory nerve study can be normal, or it can show reduced or absent SNAP amplitude.[9,11]
- Motor NCS will reveal focal slowing of ulnar motor nerve across the elbow. There should not be any slowing across the wrist or the forearm. **Fig. 4** shows an inflamed and enlarged ulnar nerve across the elbow. The speed across this compression site will be slow, but the speed of the nerve will be normal at the forearm and wrist.

What Is the Sensitivity of Electrodiagnostic Study on Ulnar Neuropathy Across the Elbow?

The sensitivity is about 50% to 80%, which is not as sensitive as EDX of CTS evaluation.[11] In addition, ulnar nerve study is technically challenging. False negative and

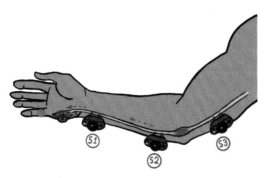

Fig. 4. Ulnar motor nerve study.

false positive results occur when there is operator error. Error on the ulnar nerve study is commonly seen on obese patients with extrasubcutaneous tissue, which makes it difficult to know the path of the ulnar nerve. Furthermore, incorrect measurements of distance can lead to wrong conclusions about velocity.

As stated before, there are many different techniques that can be used during EDX evaluation. Therefore, if the referral is for a specific disease process, such as ulnar neuropathy, this helps the electromyographer to correctly design a study to increase sensitivity. If the EDX referral does not state a specific diagnosis, then routine screening will be performed, and the diagnostic yield of the study may suffer.

What Should I Do if I Have High Clinical Suspicion of Ulnar Neuropathy Across the Elbow but the Electrodiagnostic Study Testing Result Is Normal?

In this scenario, alternative diagnoses should be considered, which include C8 radiculopathy or ulnar neuropathy across the wrist. Additional EDX testing may be needed to assess for these diagnoses.

Does my Patient Need to Have Repeat Electrodiagnostic Study After Surgical Decompression of Compressive Mononeuropathies?

If the patient's symptoms improve after surgical intervention, then repeat electrodiagnostic testing is not necessary. It is not uncommon to have continued slowing across the old compression site so repeat study will not be beneficial. If the patient's symptom returns, then repeat EDX testing should be done to check for reoccurrence of nerve entrapment. Ideally, you should have the repeat testing done with the same electromyographer so you can compare it to the prior test. Repeat tests done with the same provider will also reduce variability produced by different machine brands and different techniques used by the electromyographers.

Back and neck pain are very common problems in the elderly. There are many different medical conditions that can cause back or neck pain. A combination of musculoskeletal and neurogenic pain can occur. For diagnosis of cervical or lumbar radiculopathy, the authors commonly use the combination of history, physical examination, EDX, and imaging. Many times, the history is nonspecific, and examination is difficult to interpret because of pain, so the authors rely on EDX and imaging studies to guide them.

For example, if a patient has ipsilateral foot drop with low back pain, EDX help assess if the back pain with foot drop is caused by lumbosacral radiculopathy or by fibular (peroneal) neuropathy. Less common causes will be evaluated as well, including sciatic neuropathy or lumbosacral plexopathy. Electrodiagnostic testing will help you localize from variable sites. **Fig. 5** shows a cartoon drawing that shows potential sites of disease responsible for the patient's foot drop.

How Useful Is Electrodiagnostic Study for Diagnosis of Cervical or Lumbar Radiculopathy?

EDX is very specific in diagnosing radiculopathies. If the clinical localization and imaging levels do not match, then EDX can localize the level that is causing symptoms. This test will also search for other neurogenic cause of the patients' symptoms that may mimic radiculopathy. Last, EDX will reveal noncompressive radiculopathies when imaging is normal.

What Is the Ideal Time to Have Electrodiagnostic Study Done for a Radiculopathy?

Needle EMG is crucial for diagnosing radiculopathies. However, it takes time for Wallerian degeneration to occur before needle EMG shows the abnormalities. It is ideal to perform EMG 4 to 6 weeks after onset of symptoms.[3,9] If done earlier, findings such as spontaneous activities (positive sharp waves and fibrillations) may not be found. If the test is performed prematurely, then EMG may need to be repeated.

If the Initial Needle Electromyography Is Normal, Is There Any Utility in Repeating the Test or Performing Other Tests?

Repeating the study may be helpful. EMG has sensitivity of around 50% to 70% to detect radiculopathy. This sensitivity can be increased by sampling more muscles. For example, if you are suspecting an L5 radiculopathy, performing an EMG on multiple muscles with L5 myotomal innervation will increase the sensitivity.[12,13] Diagnoses are sometimes not initially made because of insufficient sampling of muscles. Furthermore, EMG findings change over time. Repeating a study in 3 to 6 months may reveal chronic findings that were initially not present.

If the EMG is normal, MRI would be a good complementary test. MRIs are very sensitive but have low specificity,[10] meaning there are many abnormalities on imaging that are asymptomatic. MRI and needle EMG are complementary when used together. MRI has high sensitivity, but low specificity. Needle EMG is the opposite, high in specificity but in moderate sensitivity.

What Does it Mean if MRI Is Normal, but Electromyography Indicates Radiculopathy?

In noncompressive radiculopathies, EMG will reveal physiologic abnormalities. The imaging study will be normal in noncompressive radiculopathies. Imaging studies are helpful for detecting structural abnormalities, but EMG is a dynamic test that

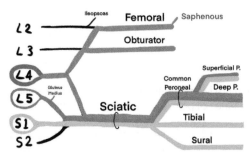

Fig. 5. Lumbosacral plexus and peripheral nerves.

reveals physiologic abnormalities. For example, varicella zoster and cytomegalovirus virus can cause infectious polyradiculitis, and MRI may not be as helpful in diagnosis.

Fibular (peroneal) neuropathy across the fibular head is a common compression site for causing foot drop in the elderly (**Fig. 6**); this could be confused for lumbar radiculopathy in patients with both foot drop and musculoskeletal back pain. The common fibular nerve is often subject to injury around the fibular head, where the nerve winds around the bone. This can occur with prolonged periods of leg crossing or be seen in hospitalized patients, where their legs are hanging off the bed and the lateral knee is pinned next to the bed railing.

Numbness and tingling in the feet

EDX is frequently ordered for symptoms of tingling and burning sensation in the feet. Tingling and burning sensation in the feet is typical early symptoms for sensory

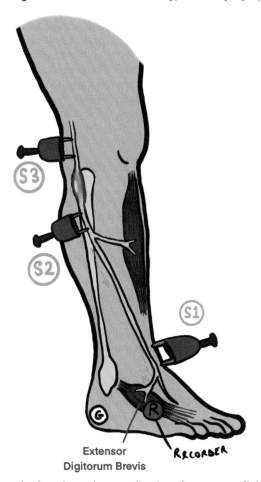

Extensor
Digitorum Brevis

RECORDER

Fig. 6. The NCS done for foot drop. The recording is at the extensor digitorum brevis muscle, and stimulation is given on the fibular nerve at the ankle, distal to the head of the fibula and proximal to the head of the fibula. On typical fibular compression neuropathy, the focal slowing (compression site) occurs between the S2 and S3 stimulation sites. The slowing here proves that the entrapment is at that site.

neuropathy, and electrodiagnostic testing can be beneficial. The goal of the electrodiagnostic testing would be to find out if the neuropathy is axonal or demyelinating in nature. The test will also tell if the neuropathy involves sensory neurons, motor neurons, or both types of fiber. The electrophysiological finding will not provide the cause of the neuropathy, but it will narrow down the potential causes for the work up. In general, there are very few primary neurologic diseases that cause neuropathy. Particularly in the elderly, neuropathy is caused by systemic disease, toxic effects from medication, and nutritional deficiency. The neuropathy is analogous to a canary in a coal mine, an early warning of toxicity.

If a patient has symmetric symptoms on both feet, a study on both legs is not necessary. Thorough evaluation in 1 leg is usually adequate for symmetric leg symptoms. The limb tested will depend on the clinical findings and may expand based on the initial findings on EDX. This will show if the neuropathy is asymmetric, length dependent, or non–length dependent. Most neuropathies are axonal in nature. Acquired demyelinating polyneuropathy requires urgent evaluation. It is typical for most electromyographers to contact the referring physician for any concerning cases.

There is an inherent problem in performing EDX on elderly patients. In this population, particularly people older than 70 years, you can find absent or reduced sural sensory nerve responses in asymptomatic people.[14] The percentage of reduced response increases with age.[14–18] If the patient does not have any neuropathic symptoms, one can mistakenly diagnose sensory neuropathy in the legs. A mistakenly diagnosed sensory neuropathy will trigger unnecessary work up and worse yet result in unwanted treatment.

Can Someone Have Neuropathy in the Feet and Have Normal Electrodiagnostic Study?

Yes, if a patient only has small sensory fiber polyneuropathy, then the electrodiagnostic testing will be normal. The NCS test only detects large fibers, and if neuropathy is isolated to only small fibers, then the testing will be normal. For example, in early diabetes, patients may present with a burning sensation in their feet, which indicates small-fiber neuropathy. In these cases, the EDX will likely be normal.

Should I Use Nerve Conduction Studies to Track Clinical Progress in my Patient with Polyneuropathy?

No, EDX is a diagnostic tool, and there is no need to repeat unless there is unexpected clinical change or concern for additional superimposed disease that was not assessed on the initial study.

What Type of Patients Should I Refer for Neurology Consult Before Ordering an Electrodiagnostic Study?

If a patient has rapidly progressive disease of unknown cause or the patient has perplexing neurologic symptoms, it would be better to consult a neurologist before EDX testing. Neurologic consultation can clarify the potential diagnosis, which will increase the yield of EDX testing.

Demyelinating polyneuropathy is a mostly immune-mediated disease that improves with treatment. If you did not suspect demyelinating disease, but the EDX report suggests demyelinating polyneuropathy, then the patient will need to see a neurologist that specializes in neuromuscular disease for urgent evaluation.

What Is the Most Common Technical Error on Electrodiagnostic Study Testing?

Performing NCS on a cold limb is arguably the most common (and most troubling) occurrence in the EMG laboratory. Performing NCS on cold hands or feet will cause slowing of nerve conduction speed, because of the normal physiologic response to cold. NCS should be done on the hands at or greater than 34°C and in the legs at or greater than 32°C.[9,19] If the test is done on cold hands or feet, patients can mistakenly get diagnosed with median neuropathy across the wrist (eg, CTS), ulnar neuropathy across the wrist, or diffuse demyelinating sensorimotor polyneuropathy (eg, GBS or CIDP). The wrong diagnosis could cause unnecessary surgery for entrapment neuropathies or treatment with immunomodulating therapies for demyelinating sensorimotor polyneuropathy. This type of error is unfortunately not uncommon (**Fig. 7**).

Age also affects the nerve conduction speed. There can be a decrease in conduction velocity of 0.5 to 4 m/s per decade.[9] This factor is amplified in older patients that are tall. A person's height has inverse correlations with nerve conduction velocity. One can mistakenly misinterpret a tall elderly person to have slow nerve conduction velocity and incorrectly diagnose demyelinating neuropathy.

There are a few steps you can take to recognize this technical error. First, if EDX impression is multiple compressive mononeuropathies or demyelinating polyneuropathy, check on the report for measured skin temperature. The NCS technician should record and report skin temperature on every EDX report. If the temperature is less than 34°C and 32°C in the hands and feet, respectively, they should warm the hands before the study. Second, if there is truly demyelinating polyneuropathy or compressive mononeuropathies, the patient should have sensory complaints and show weakness on examination. If the patient has normal reflexes and normal sensory and motor examination, then it would be safe to state that the EDX diagnosis could be wrong. This

Stim Site	NR	Peak (ms)	Norm Peak (ms)	O-P Amp (μV)	Norm O-P Amp	Dist (cm)
Right Median 2nd Antidromic Sensory (2nd Digit)						
Wrist 34.2 degrees		2.7	<3.6	64.9	>20	13.0
wrist 25.8 degrees		3.2		69.3		

Waveforms:

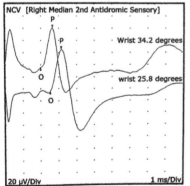

Fig. 7. The NCS of median sensory nerve study. First wave form shows normal hand temperature at 34°C, and distal peak latency is at 2.7 milliseconds. When the hand is colder than 25°C, you can see the distal peak latency is prolonged to 3.2 milliseconds. In median neuropathy across the wrist, a confirmatory finding is the prolongation of distal peak latency. Cold temperature can easily cause a false positive test result.

again illustrates that results cannot be interpreted independent of the clinical diagnosis.

SUMMARY

Electrodiagnostic testing is the primary diagnostic tool for evaluation of disease of peripheral nerve, neuromuscular junction, and muscle disease. EDX has 2 components, the NCS and needle EMG. These tests are complementary. The needle EMG is the more useful for diagnosing radiculopathy. The NCS is more useful in diagnosing entrapment neuropathies and sensorimotor polyneuropathies. NCS has relatively high sensitivity and specificity for compressive neuropathies and large-fiber sensorimotor polyneuropathies. Electrodiagnostic findings must be interpreted in context of the patient's clinical presentation. The EDX referral should have answerable questions posed to the electromyographer so that the test can be tailored to the clinical question. The EDX can provide diagnostic certainty only when used in the proper clinical context.

CLINICS CARE POINTS

- Electrodiagnostic study sensitivity is increased by electromyography referring, including clinical diagnosis, such as right carpal tunnel syndrome or left L5 radiculopathy.
- Timing is important when referring patients for electromyography evaluation for radiculopathy.
- Temperature is the most common technical error that can cause false positive test results.

DISCLOSURE

The authors have nothing to disclose.

REFERENCES

1. Martyn CN, Hughes RA. Epidemiology of peripheral neuropathy. J Neurol Neurosurg Psychiatry 1997;62:310–8.
2. Kendall R, Werner RA. Interrater reliability of the needle examination in lumbosacral radiculopathy. Muscle Nerve 2006;34:238–41.
3. Nardin RA, Raynor EM, Rutkove SB. Fibrillations in lumbosacral paraspinal muscles of normal subjects. Muscle Nerve 1998;21:1347–9.
4. Barr K. Electrodiagnosis of lumbar radiculopathy. Phys Med Rehabil Clin N Am 2013;24(1):79–91.
5. Tong HC. Specificity of needle electromyography for lumbar radiculopathy in 55- to 79-yr-old subjects with low back pain and sciatica without stenosis. Am J Phys Med Rehabil 2011;90:233–8.
6. Boon AJ, Jon TG, James CW, et al. Hematoma risk after needle electromyography. Muscle Nerve 2012;45(1):9–12.
7. AANEM. Risk in electrodiagnostic medicine. In: Guideline in electrodiagnostic medicine. Rochester (MN): American Association of Electrodiagnostic Medicine; 2014. p. P1–8.
8. Lynch SL, Boon AJ, Smith J, et al. Complications of needle electromyography: hematoma risk and correlation with anticoagulation and antiplatelet therapy. Muscle & Nerve 2008;38(4):1225–30.

9. Preston DC, Shapiro BE. Electromyography and neuromuscular disorder: clinical-electrophysiological correlations. 3rd edition. Saunders; 2012.
10. Govindarajan R, Kolb C, Salgado E. Sensitivity and specificity of MRI and EMG in diagnosing clinically evident cervical radiculopathy: a retrospective study. Neurology 2013;7(supp).
11. AANEM. Literature Review of the usefulness of nerve conduction studies and electromyography in the evaluation of patients with ulnar neuropathy at the elbow. Guidelines in electrodiagnostic medicine. American Association of Electrodiagnostic Medicine; 1996. P4-P18.
12. Dillingham TR, Pezzin LE, Lauder TD. Relationship between muscle abnormalities and symptom duration in lumbosacral radiculopathies. Am J Phys Med Rehabil 1998;77:103–7.
13. Stewart JD. Electrophysiological mapping of the segmental anatomy of the muscles of the lower extremity. Muscle Nerve 1992;15:965–6.
14. Rivner MH, Swift TR, Malik K. Influence of age and height on nerve conductions. Muscle & Nerve 2001;24(9):1134–41.
15. Dorfman LJ, Bosley TM. Age-related changes in peripheral and central nerve conduction in man. Neurology 1979;29:38–44.
16. La Fratta CW, Canestrari RE. A comparison of sensory and motor velocities as related to age. Arch Phys Med Rehabil 1966;47:286–90.
17. Bouche P, Cattelin F, Saint-Jean O, et al. Clinical and electrophysiological study of the peripheral nervous system in the elderly. J Neurol 1993;240:263–8.
18. Falco FJ, Hennessey WJ, Goldberg G, et al. Standardized nerve conduction studies in the lower limb of the healthy elderly. Am J Phys Med Rehabil 1994; 73:168–74.
19. Koo YS, Cho CS, Kim BJ. Pitfalls in using electrophysiological studies to diagnose neuromuscular disorders. J Clin Neurol 2012;8:1–14.

The Role of Imaging for Disorders of Peripheral Nerve

Natalia L. Gonzalez, MD*, Lisa D. Hobson-Webb, MD

KEYWORDS

- Nerve imaging • Nerve ultrasound • Neuromuscular ultrasound
- Nerve magnetic resolution imaging • Magnetic resolution neurography
- Focal neuropathy

KEY POINTS

- Peripheral nerve imaging is a helpful adjunct to clinical history, physical examination, and electrodiagnostic studies.
- Magnetic resolution imaging and ultrasound are used most commonly, with unique benefits and limitations for each modality and variations in use depending on local availability of expertise and equipment.
- There are no contraindications to ultrasound, and it can be performed in patients unable to lie flat and in those with pacemakers, making it particularly useful in the geriatric population.
- The role of imaging is well established in the evaluation of focal mononeuropathies, with the most common use the evaluation of compressive neuropathies.
- Advances in both ultra–high-frequency ultrasound and magnetic resolution neurography will continue to expand the applications of peripheral nerve imaging.

INTRODUCTION

The evaluation of peripheral nerve disorders historically has been limited to physical examination and electrodiagnostic studies (nerve conduction studies [NCSs] and electromyography [EMG]). Both tools primarily measure function but provide little to no anatomic information. In addition, electrodiagnostic studies may be normal in the first weeks after nerve injury. Advances in imaging technology now allow the visualization of nerves and their surrounding tissues. The clinical applications of ultrasound and magnetic resonance imaging (MRI) in peripheral nerve disorders are growing exponentially as the utility of nerve imaging becomes more apparent. This article reviews the basics of ultrasound and MRI as they relate to nerve imaging, advantages and

Department of Neurology, Neuromuscular Division, Duke University, Duke University Hospital, 3403 DUMC, Duke South Clinic 1L, Durham, NC 27710, USA
* Corresponding author.
E-mail address: natalia.gonzalez@duke.edu

Clin Geriatr Med 37 (2021) 223–239
https://doi.org/10.1016/j.cger.2021.01.001
0749-0690/21/Published by Elsevier Inc.
geriatric.theclinics.com

limitations of each imaging modality, applications of ultrasound and MRI in common neuropathies, and emerging advances in the field.

BASICS OF NERVE IMAGING
Ultrasound Basics

Ultrasonography is the practice of using sound waves to create images. The part of the system that contacts the patient directly, the transducer, sends sound waves into the tissues. It does so by converting electrical current into ultrasonic energy (piezoelectric effect). The tissue reflects some of these sounds waves back to the transducer, where they are converted into electrical signal once again. The appearance of the image is dependent on the acoustic impedance at tissue interfaces. A higher difference in densities between adjacent tissues results in greater reflection of sound waves back to the transducer and, therefore, a brighter image. Structures that appear bright, such as bone, are hyperechoic and structures that appear dark, such as fluid, are hypoechoic.

Nerve Ultrasound

Peripheral nerves vary in size but many are less than 1 mm in diameter. Therefore, high image resolution (>12 MHz) is necessary for adequate nerve visualization. This is accomplished with ultrasound in several ways. A linear array transducer, with transducer crystals oriented linearly, provides good resolution throughout the image (**Fig. 1**). A small footprint transducer can be used when imaging small and bony surfaces, such as the hands and feet, to maintain adequate contact between the surfaces of the transducer and skin. In addition to using an appropriate transducer, there are basic ultrasound system settings—power, gain, and focal zones—that can be adjusted to optimize the appearance of the nerve.

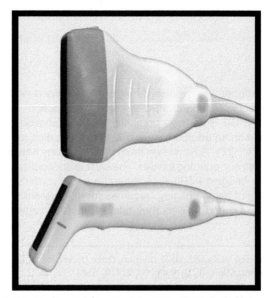

Fig. 1. Transducers commonly used for nerve imaging. Two transducers well-suited for peripheral nerve imaging are shown—a standard linear array transducer (*top*) and a footprint linear array transducer (*bottom*). The footprint transducer is preferentially used when maintaining surface contact is difficult, such as during imaging of the hands or at the elbow.

Nerves can be visualized in both cross-sectional (axial) and longitudinal views. The epineurium (outside connective tissue layer) of the nerve appears hyperechoic (bright) on ultrasound, as does the perineurium of the fascicles. This results in a honeycomb appearance on cross-sectional views and hyperechoic streaks parallel to the epineurium on longitudinal view (**Fig. 2**). Peripheral nerves typically are visualized best in the cross-sectional view and many can be traced in this way along most of their course proximally to their origins. The most commonly used parameter in the evaluation of peripheral nerves is the cross-sectional area (CSA). In general, enlargement of CSA suggests nerve compression or inflammation, whereas a reduction in CSA suggests chronic axon loss. Intraneural blood flow, which can be measured using power Doppler (**Fig. 3**), and echogenicity also often are evaluated.

Magnetic Resonance Imaging Basics

MRI utilizes differences in physical properties of protons and water molecules to distinguish between different tissues. The unique properties of water within nerves allows for use of pulse sequence techniques to dampen the surrounding tissue. T1-weighted sequences allow excellent contrast with surrounding fat and can be used to delineate nerve anatomy. T2-weighted sequences can demonstrate variations in the fluid content of the endoneurial tissue. Increased T2 signal intensity is thought to represent nerve injury due to increased blood volume and extracellular fluid in the acute or subacute phase and represent fatty infiltration in the chronic stage.[1] The addition of fat suppression to the T2-weighted sequence makes the nerves easier to image.[2] Standard MRI can show the outline of some nerves but generally is unable to distinguish nerves from similar appearing and surrounding structures. Magnetic

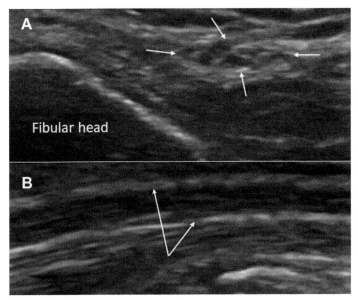

Fig. 2. (*A*) Demonstrates a normal fibular nerve (*within arrows*) visualized in the cross-sectional view at the level of the fibular head. Notice the honeycomb pattern created by the relatively hypoechoic fascicles within the nerve. (*B*) Demonstrates a median nerve at the wrist visualized in the longitudinal view. The hyperechoic epineurium lines the nerve and is well seen in this view (*arrows*).

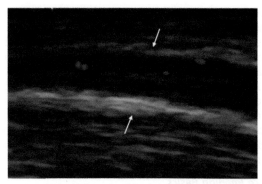

Fig. 3. Increased intraneural blood flow (*red*) is visualized in a longitudinal view of the median nerve at the wrist in a patient with carpal tunnel syndrome using power Doppler. The hyperechoic borders of the normal epineurium of the median nerve are indicated by the arrows.

resonance neurography (MRN) is a term used to describe the use of thin section and high-resolution sequences to optimize visualization of the peripheral nerves.

Magnetic Resonance Neurography

MRN initially referred to the use of diffusion-weighted and fat-suppressed pulse sequences to distinguish peripheral nerves from surrounding tissues.[3] Now, the term is used for any combination of qualitative or quantitative techniques used to image peripheral nerves. Advances in MRN have been supported by wider availability of 3T magnets and changes in surface coils that improve spatial resolution and reduce scanning time, allowing for visualization of nerve morphology, caliber, and fascicular configuration.[1,4] Three-dimensional volumetric sequences allow reformatting into curved multiplanar images along the longitudinal course of the nerve (**Fig. 4**), although

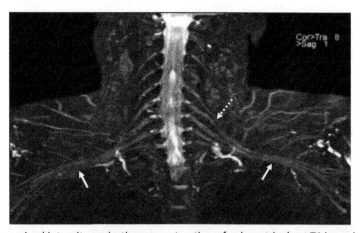

Fig. 4. A maximal intensity projection reconstruction of volumetric short T1 inversion recovery images of a normal brachial plexus is shown. The cervical nerve roots (*dotted arrow*) are well seen arising from the spinal cord and forming the brachial plexus (*solid arrows*). (*Image adapted from* Bordalo-Rodrigues M. Magnetic Resonance Neurography in Musculoskeletal Disorders. Magn Reson Imaging Clin N Am. 2018; 26(4):615-630; with permission (Figure 4 in original.).)

2-dimensional sequences carry the advantage of better spatial resolution.[1,5] Vascular suppression techniques can improve detection of small nerves, but their use remains limited by prolonged acquisition time and motion artifact.[6,7]

ULTRASOUND VERSUS MAGNETIC RESONANCE IMAGING

Ultrasound has several benefits that make it more widely used for the evaluation of peripheral nerves. It is inexpensive, easily accessible, and safe and provides high-resolution, dynamic imaging. There are no contraindications to ultrasound, and it can be performed in patients unable to lie flat, those with pacemakers, and those who suffer from claustrophobia. Because it can be performed at point of care, the examination can be altered in real time to obtain supportive information, such as comparison to a contralateral nerve. Therefore, it generally is the preferred option to image small, superficial nerves.

Ultrasound, however, does have several limitations. It is highly operator dependent and, therefore, requires experience that may not exist at a given institution. Differences among ultrasound systems limit direct comparison of images. There is a trade-off between resolution and depth of imaging; therefore, deep structures, such as the proximal sciatic nerve and lumbosacral plexus, are poorly visualized by ultrasound. Ultrasound is unable to provide an image beneath bone (eg, the brachial plexus is poorly visualized as it passes beneath the clavicle). There also is no soft tissue contrast agent at this time, limiting the detection of inflammation.

MRI provides better contrast between soft tissues and is able to image deep structures. It also is much less operator dependent, and a contrast agent (intravenous gadolinium) is widely available. The widely available MRI sequences and 1.5T scanners, however, provide poor resolution for all but the largest peripheral nerves. MRN is not yet widely available, greatly limiting its utility in most clinical practice settings.

IMAGING IN FOCAL NEUROPATHIES

Ultrasound is used most frequently in the evaluation of focal neuropathies, and, in many centers, it has become standard of practice to perform it as an adjunct to electrodiagnostic testing. Nerve imaging can be useful particularly in the evaluation of compression neuropathies (eg, carpal tunnel syndrome and ulnar neuropathy at the elbow), traumatic injury, and brachial plexopathies. In some cases, a lesion cannot be localized by using electrodiagnostic studies in isolation. Imaging may reveal focal nerve abnormalities that can confirm localization and reveal structural causes, such as traumatic neuromas, ganglion cysts, thrombosed arteries, abnormal anatomy, abscesses, or other masses.[8–10] Imaging of distal muscles can demonstrate findings of denervation and atrophy in both MRI and ultrasound, providing additional supportive information (**Fig. 5**).[11] In general, MRN is superior in detecting edema in injured nerves and can do so within 24 hours of injury, but, at this time, ultrasound provides better resolution for the assessment of size, morphologic changes and subtle fascicular distortion.[12] It also allows easy comparison to a contralateral nerve in cases of subtle abnormality or absence of an established normal reference range for the nerve of interest.

Importantly, clinical and electrodiagnostic findings in atypical causes of focal neuropathy can be similar to those found in common compression neuropathies. Therefore, imaging of the nerve should be considered in all patients presenting with focal neuropathy.

The most common and well-studied use of nerve ultrasound is the evaluation of focal compressive or entrapment neuropathies. The characteristic finding is focal

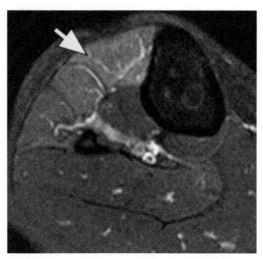

Fig. 5. An axial T2-weighted fat-suppressed image of the lower leg shows edema of the extensor muscles, including the tibilias anterior, extensor digitorum longus, and peroneus longus muscles (*arrow*), related to a fibular (peroneal) nerve compression. (*Image from* Bordalo-Rodrigues M. Magnetic Resonance Neurography in Musculoskeletal Disorders. Magn Reson Imaging Clin N Am. 2018; 26(4):615-630; with permission (Figure 6 in original.).)

enlargement of the nerve, most often just proximal to the site of compression, likely the result of edema and inflammation.[13] Other findings of nerve compression include reduced echogenicity with effacement of the normal honeycomb fascicular appearance, loss of nerve mobility, increased intraneural vascularity, and sometimes nerve flattening.[14–17] Common compressive neuropathies for which ultrasound is performed routinely include median neuropathy at the wrist (carpal tunnel syndrome), ulnar neuropathy at the elbow, radial neuropathy at the spiral groove, and fibular (peroneal) neuropathy at the fibular head. The use of ultrasound in the evaluation of carpal tunnel syndrome and ulnar neuropathy is discussed in more detail.

Carpal Tunnel Syndrome

The median nerve easily can be visualized in the cross-sectional view at the distal wrist crease, the approximate location of the carpal tunnel inlet where focal nerve enlargement is seen most frequently (**Fig. 6**). The nerve can be followed proximally into the forearm and, if needed, through its entire course up to its origin in the axilla. A wrist CSA of greater than 10 mm^2 and wrist-to-forearm CSA ratio of greater than or equal to 1.4 are highly sensitive and specific for clinical carpal tunnel syndrome when NCSs are abnormal and consistent with carpal tunnel syndrome.[14,18] Higher cutoff values of 14 mm^2 at the wrist and wrist-to-forearm ratio of greater than or equal to 1.8 can be used to diagnose CTS when clinical symptoms are present but NCSs are normal.[19,20]

Other ultrasound findings may support focal compression of the median nerve although they are difficult to quantify and therefore are more subjective. The nerve can become hypoechoic, which is visualized best in cross-section.[13,17] It also may demonstrate increased intraneural blood flow, which can be detected best with power Doppler imaging in the longitudinal view.[15] The median nerve may lose mobility and remain between the flexor retinaculum and flexor tendons during wrist flexion.[16]

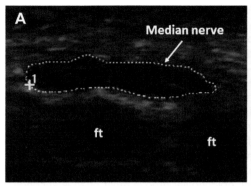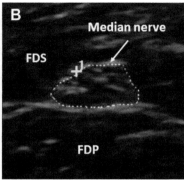

Fig. 6. Cross-sectional ultrasound images of the median nerve (A) at the wrist and (B) at the forearm are shown from a patient with carpal tunnel syndrome. At the distal wrist crease, the median nerve is hypoechoic, flattened, and enlarged with a CSA (within *dotted line*) of 18 mm² (normal ≤10 mm²). The median nerve normalizes at the mid-forearm, with a normal honeycomb pattern and CSA of 9 mm². The wrist-to-forearm ratio is 2 (normal ≤1.4), consistent with carpal tunnel syndrome. FDS, flexor digitorum superficialis muscle; FDP, flexor digitorum profundus muscle; ft, flexor tendon.

Anatomic variants, such as bifid median nerves or persistent median arteries (**Fig. 7**), can be identified by ultrasound, and documentation of their presence can be helpful for a surgeon if surgical release is pursued.[9,21]

The role of ultrasound after carpal tunnel release remains unclear, as it is with electrodiagnostic studies. Nerve enlargement may persist in asymptomatic patients after successful carpal tunnel release.[22,23] The utility of ultrasound postoperatively instead can include identifying compressive scar tissue or previously unidentified causes of the symptoms.

Ulnar Neuropathy

The ulnar nerve frequently is imaged by ultrasound in the electrodiagnostic laboratory and can be visualized along its entire course. Common regions of compression include the elbow (at the epicondylar groove or cubital tunnel) and the wrist (within Guyon

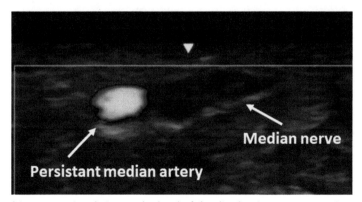

Fig. 7. In this cross-sectional view at the level of the distal wrist crease, a persistent median artery (a normal anatomic variant) easily is visualized and distinguished from the adjacent median nerve by Doppler ultrasound.

canal), and enlargement of the nerve can be at or just proximal to these sites (**Fig. 8**). Approximately 75% to 80% of lesions at the elbow are localized to the epicondylar (ulnar) groove and approximately 20% to 25% to the cubital tunnel.[24] A CSA of 10 mm^2 is used most commonly as the diagnostic cutoff value at the elbow.[25] The ulnar nerve is imaged routinely proximal to the elbow as well. It can provide a proximal CSA comparison and, rarely, it may identify ulnar nerve compression at the arcade of Struthers.[26]

A retrospective review of 64 patients with NCS/EMG confirmed ulnar neuropathy found that 25% were nonlocalizing. In these 16 patients, the addition of ultrasound aided localization of 13.[27] Even when electrodiagnostic studies are able to localize an ulnar neuropathy to the region of the elbow, more precise localization may be important for treatment planning. Ulnar neuropathy at the cubital tunnel typically is caused by entrapment and, therefore, may benefit from surgical decompression. On the other hand, ulnar neuropathy at the epicondylar groove most often is secondary to external compression or stretching due to positioning and may not benefit from surgical intervention.[28,29] Sometimes, compression can be identified at both sites.[24] Imaging may identify alternative causes of compression, including intraneural or extraneural ganglion cysts, schwannomas, anomalous anconeus epitrochlearis muscle, lymphatic malformations, abscesses, and osteophytes.[30–35]

The presence of subluxation (dislocation of the ulnar nerve over the medial epicondyle during elbow flexion) or snapping triceps (dislocation of the triceps brachii over the medial epicondyle during elbow flexion) can be identified by ultrasound. These findings may be helpful for surgical planning, but the clinical significance of their presence remains unclear.[25]

Brachial Plexopathies

The brachial plexus is a complex network of nerves connecting the cervical spinal nerve roots to the terminal upper extremity nerve branches. Causes of brachial plexopathy include trauma (such as nerve root avulsions, stretch injuries, and obstetric injuries), intrinsic and extrinsic nerve tumors, other masses, inflammatory diseases (including infection, autoimmune disease, and radiation-induced), and thoracic outlet syndrome.

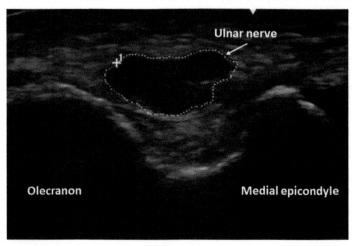

Fig. 8. Demonstrated is a cross-sectional view of an ulnar nerve at the medial epicondylar (ulnar) groove in a patient with ulnar neuropathy. The ulnar nerve is hypoechoic and focally enlarged at this site, with a CSA (within the *dotted line*) of 27 mm^2 (normal <10 mm^2).

Ultrasound commonly is used for the evaluation of brachial plexopathies. It has the advantage of providing dynamic imaging to evaluate for compression during abduction or external rotation in cases of thoracic outlet syndrome.[36] It also is particularly good for assessing nerve sheath tumors and perineural fibrosis.[37]

Ultrasound of the brachial plexus, however, requires an operator with technical expertise, and imaging is interrupted in the costoclavicular region due to bone shadowing. For this reason, MRI plays an important role in evaluation of the brachial plexus, and MRN is particularly useful for visualization of nerve discontinuity or root avulsion. Gadolinium contrast can be used when evaluating for neoplastic and inflammatory causes. For example, an inflammatory plexopathy can occur following radiation treatment, and MRI can be used to distinguish this from tumor recurrence.

Traumatic Neuropathies

A major limitation of electrodiagnostic studies for the evaluation of nerve trauma is the delay in which abnormalities are detected, often at least several weeks following injury. Even after the changes occur, it may be difficult to distinguish partial from complete transections. Months may pass before this becomes apparent, delaying surgical repair, which has been shown to result in poor outcomes.[38] Therefore, imaging can play an important role in traumatic nerve lesions, and ultrasound is particularly helpful by providing dynamic images from different angles.[39] MRN may be preferred in the assessment of deeper nerves, as discussed previously, because edema in injured nerve may be seen as T2 hyperintensity as early as 24 hours after injury.[12] In a retrospective review of 143 patients with suspected traumatic peripheral nerve lesions, ultrasound was most useful when electrodiagnostic findings were severe after acute trauma and suggested nerve transection. In these cases, ultrasound was able to distinguish complete from partial nerve transections. It was less likely to be helpful in cases of only mild, demyelinating electrodiagnostic changes after blunt trauma.[40] In addition to providing information about the continuity of a nerve, imaging can identify anatomic changes, the presence of tandem lesions, the position of proximal and distal nerve stumps, bony compression, pseudoaneurysms, and, more chronically, neuromas and fibrosis (**Fig. 9**).[38] These findings are helpful for orientation and planning of a surgical intervention.[41]

CASE 1: A COMMON CLINICAL QUERY—IS THIS A CASE OF FIBULAR NEUROPATHY OR L5 RADICULOPATHY?
Case Presentation

A 77-year-old man with a history of L5-S1 laminectomy presented with 3 months of pain in the right lower extremity in the setting of worsening back pain. On physical examination, there was weakness of right ankle dorsiflexion and eversion, decreased pinprick sensation over the dorsal foot and lateral lower leg with intact reflexes in the lower extremities. NCSs demonstrated reduced amplitudes of the right fibular motor responses to the extensor digitorum brevis and tibialis anterior muscles, a prolonged right fibular F-wave latency, and a borderline reduced right superficial fibular sensory response amplitude. Needle examination demonstrated evidence of active denervation and chronic reinnervation in the right tibialis anterior and peroneus longus muscles.

Clinical Questions and Discussion

Do the electrodiagnostic findings definitively localize the lesion?
The major findings from the NCSs were reduced amplitudes of the fibular motor responses and a prolonged fibular F-wave latency. These findings could be seen either

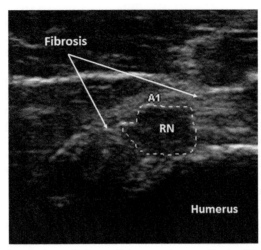

Fig. 9. A cross-sectional view of the radial nerve in a patient with radial nerve palsy following a comminuted fracture of the humerus is shown. The radial nerve (RN), shown within the dotted line, is focally enlarged with a CSA of 21 mm² (normal ≤10 mm²) and surrounded by fibrosis (arrows), demonstrated on ultrasound as hypoechoic streaks.

in focal fibular neuropathy or predominantly L5 radiculopathy. Abnormality of the superficial fibular sensory response suggests a common fibular neuropathy, but this is a technically difficult nerve to study and, in this case, there was only a borderline reduction in amplitude. The needle examination results were supportive of a common fibular neuropathy in the region of the knee. Given the clinical history of degenerative disease of the lower lumbar spine, however, report of concomitant back pain, absence of focal slowing of the fibular response across the knee, and relatively preserved superficial fibular sensory response, a more conclusive study was desired.

Is there a role for nerve imaging in this case?
Yes. Ultrasound was readily available in the laboratory and performed at the time of the electrodiagnostic study (**Fig. 10**). Focal enlargement of the fibular nerve was seen at the level of the fibular head, with the CSA measuring 22 mm² (normal ≤12 mm²). These findings confirmed a focal common fibular neuropathy at the fibular head, a common site of compression. This was supported further by reduced echogenicity and a mild increase in intraneural blood flow. Importantly, there was no evidence of a structural cause that would alter the plan for this patient's management. For example, structural causes of common fibular neuropathy include intraneural ganglion cysts, lipomas, and abnormal biceps femoris anatomy.[42–44]

IMAGING IN GENERALIZED NEUROPATHIES
Hereditary and Acquired Inflammatory Demyelinating Neuropathies

Ultrasound also has utility in the diagnosis of some generalized peripheral neuropathies, particularly when NCSs are inconclusive; when an underlying polyneuropathy, such as from diabetes mellitus, makes differentiation of a separate process difficult; or when the severity of the neuropathy makes it difficult to distinguish demyelinating from axonal features using electrodiagnostic studies alone. Ultrasound is most useful in cases of demyelinating polyneuropathies, which are characterized by nerve enlargement that can occur anywhere along the course of the nerve. In hereditary demyelinating neuropathies (eg, Charcot-Marie-Tooth [CMT] type 1a), nerve enlargement is

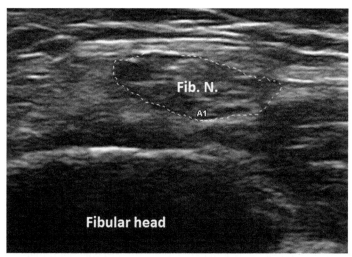

Fig. 10. An ultrasound image from case 1 is shown. The fibular nerve (Fib. N.), with its border outlined by the dotted line "A1", is focally enlarged at the fibular head, with a CSA of 22 mm² (normal ≤12 mm²).

diffuse, whereas in acquired inflammatory polyneuropathies, such as chronic inflammatory demyelinating polyradiculoneuropathy (CIDP), multifocal motor neuropathy (MMN), and Guillain-Barré syndrome (GBS), nerve enlargement is multifocal.

In CIDP, focal nerve enlargement at noncompressible sites is seen most commonly in the proximal upper extremities.[45] Nerve imaging is particularly valuable in CIDP because it can be difficult to capture conduction block in these proximal regions using NCSs alone. Focal nerve enlargement also can be seen in the cervical spinal nerve roots and brachial plexus; in these regions, ultrasound has demonstrated similar sensitivity to MRI in both MMN and CIDP.[46] Although there is consideration of adding ultrasound to the diagnostic criteria for CIDP, diagnosis of CIDP is made primarily based on clinical history and electrodiagnostic findings at this time.[47] The current diagnostic criteria for CIDP do, however, include enlargement or gadolinium enhancement on MRI of the spinal roots, brachial plexus, or lumbosacral plexus as a supportive criterion.[47]

The role of ultrasound in the diagnosis of GBS still is not well defined, but some patients with GBS have enlargement of peripheral nerves.[48,49] There may be a unique role for ultrasound in the diagnosis of GBS because NCSs may be normal or demonstrate only subtle abnormalities during the first 2 weeks.[50]

Other Polyneuropathies

Nerve imaging is less useful for axonal neuropathies, which typically demonstrate either mild or no nerve enlargement.[51] Diabetic polyneuropathy typically is a mixed demyelinating and axonal polyneuropathy and commonly associated with mild peripheral nerve enlargement, but for now, there is no role for the use of nerve imaging in the diagnosis of diabetic polyneuropathy.[52] Nerve ultrasound may be helpful in the evaluation of other rare neuropathies, such as leprosy and vasculitic neuropathy.[53,54]

CASE 2: A CASE OF LOWER EXTREMITY BURNING PAIN AND URINARY INCONTINENCE
Case Presentation

A 72-year-old woman presented with several years of lower greater than upper extremity burning dysesthesias, back and radicular pain, and urinary incontinence. On examination, strength was normal, but vibration, pinprick, and proprioception were reduced below the knees with absent Achilles reflexes. EMG/NCS was notable only for absent sural responses. Cerebrospinal fluid protein was elevated at 173 mg/dL, supportive of a diagnosis of chronic immune sensory polyradiculopathy (CISP), an atypical sensory variant of CIDP.

Clinical Questions and Discussion

Does the diagnosis of chronic immune sensory polyradiculopathy explain this patient's symptoms?

Not fully. CISP would not explain urinary incontinence, which typically localizes to the central rather than peripheral nervous system.

Does nerve imaging play a role in this case?

Yes. In this case, the region of interest was the lumbosacral spine. First, cauda equina syndrome remained a concern. Second, CIDP and CIDP variants are inflammatory radiculoneuropathies, and their diagnosis can be supported by enlargement and sometimes contrast enhancement of nerve roots. An MRI was performed. Ultrasound would be a poor choice in this case, given the depth and amount of bone artifact in the area of interest and lack of a contrast agent.

MRI demonstrated enlarged, contrast-enhancing lumbosacral nerve roots, which supported the diagnosis of a CIDP variant (**Fig. 11**). In addition, these massively enlarged nerve roots appeared compressed within the spinal canal. The patient underwent decompressive laminectomy with partial improvement in sensory symptoms and resolution of urinary incontinence.

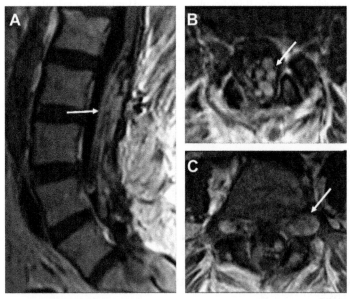

Fig. 11. MRIs with and without contrast of the lumbosacral spine from case 2 are shown. T1 flair MRI demonstrates contrast-enhancing, enlarged, cauda equina nerve roots (arrows), seen in (A) sagittal and (B) axial views. (C) Enlarged S1 nerve roots are seen exiting the neural foramen in an axial view (arrow).

FUTURE DIRECTIONS

Emerging technologies in ultrasound have the potential to improve several existing limitations in the use of ultrasound for peripheral nerve imaging.[55] Ultra–high-frequency transducers (>22 MHz) now are commercially available and can provide detailed images of superficial nerves, including individual nerve fascicles. Photoacoustic imaging can improve the morphologic view of nerves, whereas shear wave elastography can provide a measure of tissue stiffness.

The utility of MRN in the clinical setting will continue to grow as the availability of improved magnet and coil technology and advanced software expands. New and improved technologies will improve the quality of peripheral nerve evaluation further, including software advances to reduce respiratory motion artifact and advances in diffusion-weighted imaging to assess directionality and magnitude of diffusion to provide more quantitative evaluation of nerve injury.[2,12] Applications of artificial intelligence have the potential to advance optimization of both MRI and ultrasound imaging and interpretation. Finally, in addition to improvements in technology and software, research in the clinical applications of nerve imaging is growing rapidly and will continue to expand the evidence-based use of nerve imaging in the clinic as well as in the clinical trial setting.

SUMMARY

The evaluation of disorders of the peripheral nerve often requires a multifaceted approach. Clinical history, physical examination, and electrodiagnostic studies provide essential information regarding function and often localization of nerve injury. For focal neuropathies, in particular, nerve imaging can be a valuable and sometimes essential adjunct, providing precise anatomic localization and sometimes identifying an unexpected structural cause. Imaging in the evaluation of generalized neuropathies is a growing field with the utility of nerve imaging most well-established in the diagnosis of acquired inflammatory polyneuropathies, particularly in CIDP.

Ultrasound and MRI are commonly used imaging modalities for nerve pathology, and each has its own set of benefits and limitations. In general, ultrasound is used more commonly because it is safe, widely available, and inexpensive and provides high-resolution, dynamic imaging that can be obtained at point of care. MRI, in particular MRN, however, generally is better suited for the evaluation of acute trauma, nerves that are deep or surrounded by bony structures, and situations in which use of a tissue contrast agent may be beneficial. It also is much less operator dependent. Local availability of equipment and expertise often influences patterns of use. Regardless, applications for each modality will continue to expand with advances in technology.

CLINICS CARE POINTS

- Ultrasound is used more commonly for peripheral nerve imaging because it is safe, inexpensive, and provides high-resolution, dynamic imaging that can be obtained at point of care. MRN is better suited for the evaluation of acute trauma, nerves that are deep or surrounded by bony structures, and tumors in which use of a tissue contrast agent may be beneficial.

- Clinical and electrodiagnostic findings in atypical causes of focal neuropathy can be similar to those found in common compression neuropathies. Unexpected structural etiologies, such as ganglion cysts, lipomas, or pseudoaneurysms, may be present and identified only if imaging is pursued. Nerve imaging should be considered in all patients presenting with focal neuropathy.

- Characteristic ultrasound findings of compressive or entrapment neuropathies include focal enlargement just proximal to the site of compression, reduced echogenicity, and increase intraneural vascularity.
- Imaging abnormalities may be present even when nerve conduction abnormalities are absent. This is well established in carpal tunnel syndrome.
- Even when electrodiagnostic studies are able to localize an ulnar neuropathy to the region of the elbow, more precise localization can be important in surgical planning.
- Peripheral nerve imaging plays a major role in trauma because electrodiagnostic changes may not be present for several weeks.
- Nerve imaging can be used as an adjunct in the diagnosis of acquired inflammatory polyneuropathies, in particular, CIDP.

DISCLOSURE

The authors have nothing to disclose.

REFERENCES

1. Bordalo-Rodrigues M. Magnetic resonance neurography in musculoskeletal disorders. Magn Reson Imaging Clin N Am 2018;26:615–30.
2. Sneag DB, Queler S. Technological advancements in magnetic resonance neurography. Curr Neurol Neurosci Rep 2019;19:75.
3. Sneag DB, Rancy SK, Wolfe SW, et al. Brachial plexitis or neuritis? MRI features of lesion distribution in Parsonage-Turner syndrome. Muscle Nerve 2018;58:359–66.
4. Martín Noguerol T, Barousse R, Socolovsky M, et al. Quantitative magnetic resonance (MR) neurography for evaluation of peripheral nerves and plexus injuries. Quant Imaging Med Surg 2017;7:398–421.
5. Balsiger F, Steindel C, Arn M, et al. Segmentation of peripheral nerves from magnetic resonance neurography: a fully-automatic, deep learning-based approach. Front Neurol 2018;9:777.
6. Cervantes B, Kirschke JS, Klupp E, et al. Orthogonally combined motion- and diffusion-sensitized driven equilibrium (OC-MDSDE) preparation for vessel signal suppression in 3D turbo spin echo imaging of peripheral nerves in the extremities. Magn Reson Med 2018;79:407–15.
7. Yoneyama M, Takahara T, Kwee TC, et al. Rapid high resolution MR neurography with a diffusion-weighted pre-pulse. Magn Reson Med Sci 2013;12:111–9.
8. Hobson-Webb LD, Walker FO. Traumatic neuroma diagnosed by ultrasonography. Arch Neurol 2004;61:1322–3.
9. Padua L, Di Pasquale A, Liotta G, et al. Ultrasound as a useful tool in the diagnosis and management of traumatic nerve lesions. Clin Neurophysiol 2013;124:1237–43.
10. Kele H, Verheggen R, Reimers CD. Carpal tunnel syndrome caused by thrombosis of the median artery: importance of high-resolution ultrasonography for diagnosis: case report. J Neurosurg 2002;97:471–3.
11. Hobson-Webb LD, Massey JM, Juel VC, et al. The ultrasonographic wrist-to-forearm median nerve area ratio in carpal tunnel syndrome. Clin Neurophysiol 2008;119:1353–7.
12. Holzgrefe RE, Wagner ER, Singer AD, et al. Imaging of the peripheral nerve: concepts and future direction of magnetic resonance neurography and ultrasound. J Hand Surg Am 2019;44:1066–79.

13. Cartwright MS, White DL, Demar S, et al. Median nerve changes following steroid injection for carpal tunnel syndrome. Muscle Nerve 2011;44:25–9.

14. Fowler JR, Munsch M, Tosti R, et al. Comparison of ultrasound and electrodiagnostic testing for diagnosis of carpal tunnel syndrome: study using a validated clinical tool as the reference standard. J Bone Joint Surg Am 2014;96:e148.

15. Mallouhi A, Pültzl P, Trieb T, et al. Predictors of carpal tunnel syndrome: accuracy of gray-scale and color Doppler sonography. AJR Am J Roentgenol 2006;186: 1240–5.

16. Nakamichi K, Tachibana S. Restricted motion of the median nerve in carpal tunnel syndrome. J Hand Surg 2016. https://doi.org/10.1016/S0266-7681(05)80153-6.

17. Tai T-W, Wu C-Y, Su F-C, et al. Ultrasonography for diagnosing carpal tunnel syndrome: a meta-analysis of diagnostic test accuracy. Ultrasound Med Biol 2012; 38:1121–8.

18. Mhoon JT, Juel VC, Hobson-Webb LD. Median nerve ultrasound as a screening tool in carpal tunnel syndrome: Correlation of cross-sectional area measures with electrodiagnostic abnormality. Muscle Nerve 2012;46:861–70.

19. Billakota S, Hobson-Webb LD. Standard median nerve ultrasound in carpal tunnel syndrome: a retrospective review of 1,021 cases. Clin Neurophysiol Pract 2017;2:188–91.

20. Aseem F, Williams JW, Walker FO, et al. Neuromuscular ultrasound in patients with carpal tunnel syndrome and normal nerve conduction studies. Muscle Nerve 2017;55:913–5.

21. Bayrak IK, Bayrak AO, Kale M, et al. Bifid median nerve in patients with carpal tunnel syndrome. J Ultrasound Med 2008;27:1129–36.

22. Smidt MH, Visser LH. Carpal tunnel syndrome: clinical and sonographic follow-up after surgery. Muscle Nerve 2008;38:987–91.

23. Vögelin E, Nüesch E, Jüni P, et al. Sonographic follow-up of patients with carpal tunnel syndrome undergoing surgical or nonsurgical treatment: prospective cohort study. J Hand Surg Am 2010;35:1401–9.

24. Omejec G, Podnar S. Precise localization of ulnar neuropathy at the elbow. Clin Neurophysiol 2015;126:2390–6.

25. Beekman R, Visser LH, Verhagen WI. Ultrasonography in ulnar neuropathy at the elbow: a critical review. Muscle Nerve 2011;43:627–35.

26. Sivak WN, Hagerty SE, Huyhn L, et al. Diagnosis of ulnar nerve entrapment at the arcade of Struthers with electromyography and ultrasound. Plast Reconstr Surg Glob Open 2016;4:e648.

27. Pelosi L, Tse DMY, Mulroy E, et al. Ulnar neuropathy with abnormal non-localizing electrophysiology: clinical, electrophysiological and ultrasound findings. Clin Neurophysiol 2018;129:2155–61.

28. Omejec G, Podnar S. What causes ulnar neuropathy at the elbow? Clin Neurophysiol 2016;127:919–24.

29. Simon NG. Treatment of ulnar neuropathy at the elbow - an ongoing conundrum. Clin Neurophysiol 2018;129:1716–7.

30. Chang WK, Li YP, Zhang DF, et al. The cubital tunnel syndrome caused by the intraneural or extraneural ganglion cysts: case report and review of the literature. J Plast Reconstr Aesthet Surg 2017;70:1404–8.

31. Dekelver I, Van Glabbeek F, Dijs H, et al. Bilateral ulnar nerve entrapment by the M. anconeus epitrochlearis. A case report and literature review. Clin Rheumatol 2012;31:1139–42.

32. Filippou G, Mondelli M, Greco G, et al. Ulnar neuropathy at the elbow: how frequent is the idiopathic form? An ultrasonographic study in a cohort of patients. Clin Exp Rheumatol 2010;28:63–7.
33. Liu MT, Lee JT, Wang CH, et al. Cubital tunnel syndrome caused by ulnar nerve schwannoma in a patient with diabetic sensorimotor polyneuropathy. Acta Neurol Taiwan 2016;25:60–4.
34. Lugão HB, Frade MAC, Mazzer N, et al. Leprosy with ulnar nerve abscess: ultrasound findings in a child. Skeletal Radiol 2017;46:137–40.
35. González Pérez I, Corella Montoya F, Casado Fariñas I. Intraneural microcystic lymphatic malformation of the ulnar nerve at the Guyon canal: unusual cause of ulnar pain in a child. Orthop Traumatol Surg Res 2017;103:513–5.
36. Demondion X, Herbinet P, Boutry N, et al. Sonographic mapping of the normal brachial plexus. Am J Neuroradiol 2003;24:1303–9.
37. Griffith JF. Ultrasound of the brachial plexus. Semin Musculoskelet Radiol 2018; 22:323–33.
38. Tagliafico A, Altafini L, Garello I, et al. Traumatic neuropathies: spectrum of imaging findings and postoperative assessment. Semin Musculoskelet Radiol 2010; 14:512–22.
39. Cartwright MS, Yoon JS, Lee KH, et al. Diagnostic ultrasound for traumatic radial neuropathy. Am J Phys Med Rehabil 2011;90:342–3.
40. Omejec G, Podnar S. Contribution of ultrasonography in evaluating traumatic lesions of the peripheral nerves. Neurophysiol Clin 2020;50(2):93–101.
41. Cokluk C, Aydin K, Senel A. Presurgical ultrasound-assisted neuro-examination in the surgical repair of peripheral nerve injury. Minim Invasive Neurosurg 2004;47: 169–72.
42. Cartwright MS, Passmore LV, Yoon J-S, et al. Cross-sectional area reference values for nerve ultrasonography. Muscle Nerve 2008;37:566–71.
43. Grant TH, Omar IM, Dumanian GA, et al. Sonographic evaluation of common peroneal neuropathy in patients with foot drop. J Ultrasound Med 2015;34: 705–11.
44. Visser LH. High-resolution sonography of the common peroneal nerve: detection of intraneural ganglia. Neurology 2006;67:1473–5.
45. Scheidl E, Böhm J, Simó M, et al. Different patterns of nerve enlargement in polyneuropathy subtypes as detected by ultrasonography. Ultrasound Med Biol 2014; 40:1138–45.
46. Goedee HS, Jongbloed BA, van Asseldonk J-TH, et al. A comparative study of brachial plexus sonography and magnetic resonance imaging in chronic inflammatory demyelinating neuropathy and multifocal motor neuropathy. Eur J Neurol 2017;24:1307–13.
47. Joint Task Force of the EFNS and the PNS. European Federation of Neurological societies/peripheral nerve society guideline on management of multifocal motor neuropathy. Report of a joint task force of the European Federation of Neurological societies and the peripheral nerve society–first revision. J Peripher Nerv Syst 2010;15:295–301.
48. Kerasnoudis A, Tsivgoulis G. Nerve ultrasound in peripheral neuropathies: a review. J Neuroimaging 2015;25:528–38.
49. Zaidman CM, Harms MB, Pestronk A. Ultrasound of inherited vs. acquired demyelinating polyneuropathies. J Neurol 2013;260:3115–21.
50. Gordon PH, Wilbourn AJ. Early electrodiagnostic findings in Guillain-Barré syndrome. Arch Neurol 2001;58:913–7.

51. Telleman JA, Grimm A, Goedee S, et al. Nerve ultrasound in polyneuropathies. Muscle Nerve 2018;57:716–28.
52. Breiner A, Qrimli M, Ebadi H, et al. Peripheral nerve high-resolution ultrasound in diabetes. Muscle Nerve 2017;55:171–8.
53. Grimm A, Décard BF, Bischof A, et al. Ultrasound of the peripheral nerves in systemic vasculitic neuropathies. J Neurol Sci 2014;347:44–9.
54. Martinoli C, Derchi LE, Bertolotto M, et al. US and MR imaging of peripheral nerves in leprosy. Skeletal Radiol 2000;29:142–50.
55. Hobson-Webb LD. Emerging technologies in neuromuscular ultrasound. Muscle Nerve 2020;61:719–25.

Common Compression Neuropathies

Svetlana Faktorovich, MD[a,b,]*, Asia Filatov, MD[a,b], Zufe Rizvi, MD[a,b]

KEYWORDS

- Compression neuropathy • Entrapment neuropathy • Carpal tunnel syndrome
- Cubital tunnel syndrome • Foot drop

KEY POINTS

- Compression neuropathies present with weakness and sensory changes in the distribution of the affected nerve.
- For mild to moderate compression neuropathies, conservative management should be considered initially.
- In moderate to severe cases, or in those refractory to conservative therapy, surgery should be considered.
- Conservative therapy includes stabilizing the associated joint, splinting, and avoiding triggering activities. Clinicians should spend the time to educate their patients on how to do so appropriately.

COMMON COMPRESSION MONONEUROPATHIES

Entrapment mononeuropathies, also known as compression neuropathies, are common neurologic conditions resulting in pain, numbness, and weakness in the distribution of the affected nerve. They occur most often occur as a result of mechanical injury, such as from direct compression or stretch, as the affected nerve travels through a distinct anatomic space, such as a narrow fibrous or osseous tissue. As a result, the nerve undergoes demyelinating changes and impaired signal transmission. If left untreated, these conditions can result in long-term axonal damage and disability. Compression neuropathies are common in the adult population and are a common reason for referral for electromyography (EMG)/nerve conduction studies (NCS).[1] This article explores cases of nontraumatic and common compression mononeuropathies and their clinical presentations.

Funding & Conflict of Interest: None.
[a] Florida Atlantic University, Charles E. Schmidt College of Medicine, Boca Raton, FL, USA;
[b] Marcus Neuroscience Institute, Boca Raton Regional Hospital, 800 Meadow Road, Boca Raton, FL 33486, USA
* Corresponding author.
E-mail address: sfaktorovich@baptisthealth.net

COMPRESSION MONONEUROPATHIES
Median Neuropathy at the Carpal Tunnel

Carpal tunnel syndrome (CTS) is the most common form of entrapment neuropathy. It arises as a result of median nerve entrapment as it crosses under the flexor retinaculum, also known as the transverse carpal ligament, a fibrous band at the base of the palm. Along with the adjacent carpal bones, this fibrous tissue forms the border of the carpal tunnel, after which the condition is named. This is illustrated in **Fig. 1**.

CTS typically is a slowly progressive condition, seen more often in women than in men. Initially, symptoms typically are intermittent, provoked by activities involving hyperflexion/hyperextension of the wrist, such as doing yoga or pushups, typing on a computer, and using a steering wheel. Symptoms often are more pronounced at night. CTS often is bilateral, although it tends to be more severe in the dominant hand. Physical examination often shows median distribution sensory loss in digits 1 to 3 at the palm with thenar sparing (**Fig. 2**). In more severe cases, weakness and atrophy of the abductor pollicis brevis muscle are common findings. Tapping over the carpal tunnel often elicits symptoms, known as Tinel sign. Another common test, known as the Phalen maneuver, involves having the patient forcibly flex the wrists for up to 1 minute and monitoring for symptom exacerbation. If positive, this also

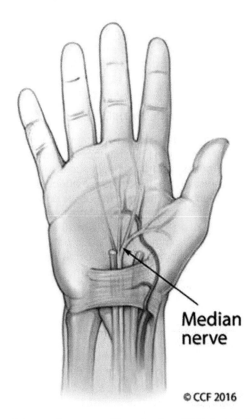

Median nerve

© CCF 2016

Fig. 1. Compression of the median nerve. (*From* Gardner BT, Dale AM, Buckner-petty S, et al. Functional measures developed for clinical populations identified impairment among active workers with upper extremity disorders. *J Occup Rehabil.* 2016;26(1):84-94.)

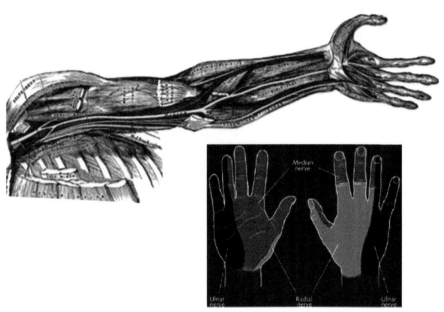

Fig. 2. Median nerve. (*From* Murphy KA, Morrisonponce D. Anatomy, Shoulder and Upper Limb, Median Nerve. [Updated 2020 Jul 31]. In: StatPearls [Internet]. Treasure Island (FL): StatPearls Publishing; 2020 Jan-. Available from: https://www.ncbi.nlm.nih.gov/books/NBK448084/.)

can suggest the presence of CTS. Even though the sensory distribution of the median nerve involves only the first 4 digits, patient with CTS may complain of sensory symptoms and pain in all 5 fingers, the rest of the hand and occasionally the symptoms can ascend above the level of the wrist. EMG/NCS is effective in confirming the diagnosis and determining the severity.

Although usually a slowly progressive condition, CTS can present acutely, typically after a distal radius fracture.[2] It also has been described as a rare side effect of checkpoint inhibitors, a category of immunotherapy used in cancer treatment that has been associated with a wide range of autoimmune conditions.[3] Additional rare causes include local hemorrhage and vascular disorders. In the acute setting, EMG/NCS testing has limited sensitivity, and diagnosis of CTS relies on clinical history and examination. EMG/NCS studies within the first week may show early nerve injury; however, severity and prognosis cannot be determined without assessing the degree of axonal injury, which can become apparent at approximately 10 days to 4 weeks following the initial event.[4]

Multiple predispositions exist for the development of CTS, including but not limited to diabetes, pregnancy, and thyroid dysfunction, among others, as detailed in **Table 1**. An atypical etiology for CTS beyond repetitive use should be considered particularly if a patient develops symptoms and nerve dysfunction in the nondominant hand. Mild to moderate cases of CTS initially can be managed conservatively (wrist splint, avoiding provoking activities, or ergonomic devices). In more severe cases, however, local steroid injection and surgical nerve release often are necessary. Clinically significant weakness in the median-innervated muscles of the hand should warrant prompt surgical evaluation, even at the time of diagnosis.

Table 1 Etiologies of carpal tunnel syndrome	
Repetitive maneuvers	Trauma
Obesity	Mass lesions
Pregnancy	Amyloidosis
Arthritis	Sarcoidosis
Hypothyroidism	Multiple myeloma
Diabetes mellitus	Leukemia

Note: etiologies are listed in approximate order of most to least common.

Predisposing condition: compression of the median nerve. *From* Gardner BT, Dale AM, Buckner-petty S, et al. Functional measures developed for clinical populations identified impairment among active workers with upper extremity disorders. *J Occup Rehabil.* 2016;26(1):84-94.

Ulnar Neuropathy at the Elbow

Ulnar neuropathy is another common mononeuropathy, both acutely after elbow trauma and in the event of a chronic compression neuropathy. Entrapment occurs most often due to mechanical compression or stretch of the nerve at the ulnar groove at the elbow, where it lies superficially, or within the cubital tunnel, an anatomic space formed by the heads of the flexor carpi ulnaris muscle, underneath the Osborne ligament.[5] These patients often complain of tingling and numbness in the ulnar distribution of the hand, including the fourth and fifth digits and medial side of the palm (see **Fig. 2**). Initially, the symptoms occur intermittently, often worse at night or during sustained elbow flexion. As the condition progresses, symptoms become more frequent, eventually resulting in intrinsic hand muscle weakness and wasting as well as weakness of the ulnar-innervated forearm muscles. Froment sign is a characteristic finding, due to adductor pollicis (AP) weakness (**Fig. 3**). When a patient is asked to pinch a piece of paper, the median-innervated flexor pollicis longus and flexor digitorum profundus muscles contract to compensate for AP weakness, resulting in flexion of the thumb and index finger. Common exacerbating activities include driving and leaning on the affected elbow. Professions that involve overuse of the elbow joint, such as manual labor or athletics that involve excessive throwing (eg, baseball), have an increased

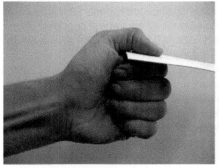 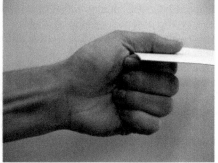

Fig. 3. Froment sign. (*From* Goldman SB, Brininger TL, Schrader JW. A Review of Clinical Tests and Signs for the Assessment of Ulnar Neuropathy. J Hand Ther, 2009; 22 (3): 209-220.)

risk of ulnar neuropathy. Those individuals often develop concurrent, overuse-related bony and soft tissue disease at the elbow joint, such as ligamentous instability, medial epicondylitis, and stress fractures, among others.[5] Ganglion cysts, tumors, history of elbow fracture, secondary arthritic changes (tardy ulnar palsy), and elbow fractures also can trigger ulnar neuropathy.

The wrist is another common site for ulnar nerve compression. People who apply extended pressure on the hypothenar eminence, such as cyclists and laborers from drilling activities, are at a greater risk for compression of the ulnar nerve located at Guyon canal, a space formed proximally by the pisiform bone and distally by the hook of the hamate.[6] This results in an injury to the deep motor branch of the ulnar nerve as it travels through the Guyon canal, leading to weakness and wasting of the ulnar intrinsic hand muscles, similar to that seen with ulnar entrapment at the elbow. This lesion, however, often is painless and without sensory disturbance, given sparing of the superficial, sensory branch. In addition, ulnar-innervated forearm muscle are spared.

Management of an ulnar compression neuropathy depends on severity. Conservative therapy should be used initially in the setting of mild cases. The patient should be educated on provoking factors, including elbow positioning and activity modification, to minimize stretch or compression of the ulnar nerve if compression is located at the elbow. For example, hyperflexion of the elbow (such as during sleep) and leaning the elbow against a hard surface should be avoided. Additionally, patients can consider the use of protective soft padding, such as a towel, wrapped over the elbow at night. Rigid splinting is another effective alternative.[7] Surgical nerve release should be considered in cases of moderate to severe neuropathy or when conservative therapy fails. If a patient presents with significant intrinsic hand weakness, surgery should be considered at the time of presentation.

Radial Neuropathy

Radial nerve injuries are seen less commonly than median and ulnar neuropathies. Radial nerve entrapment can occur at various points along the nerve's course, such as the main trunk in the proximal arm or isolated branches of the nerve distally. The most common site of entrapment is at the site of the spiral groove in the upper arm, where the nerve lies along the humerus, making it susceptible to compression. For example, this can occur during surgery if the nerve is compressed at the humerus against the operating table or from prolonged tightening of an arterial pressure cuff. Symptoms typically include burning pain, numbness, and paresthesias at the dorsal surface of the hand, sometimes extending above the wrist, as well as weakness in radial-innervated muscles. Physical examination includes wrist and finger drop due to weakness in wrist extensors and finger extensors, sparing the wrist and finger flexors. In addition, brachioradialis weakness and reduced deep tendon reflex often are seen. Triceps reflex and motor strength characteristically are spared with injuries at the spiral groove, as its motor fibers are given off proximal to the spiral groove. **Fig. 4** provides an illustration of radial nerve injury in different sections including the radial groove and the axilla.

If entrapment at the spiral groove is suspected without a known trigger, imaging should be done to look for the source of compression, such as a tumor, cyst, or humeral fracture. Initial treatment of radial nerve injury at the spinal groove often is treated with rest, immobilization, and neuropathic pain medication, as needed. Prolonged immobilization, however, is not recommended. Surgery may be indicated in the case of nerve transection, open fracture, or failure of conservative therapy.

Radial nerve injury also can be seen at the level of the axilla. If compressed at this level, triceps weakness and loss of triceps deep tendon reflex are seen, in addition to

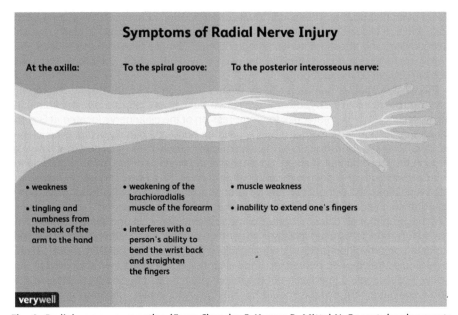

Symptoms of Radial Nerve Injury

At the axilla:
To the spiral groove:
To the posterior interosseous nerve:

- weakness
- tingling and numbness from the back of the arm to the hand

- weakening of the brachioradialis muscle of the forearm
- interferes with a person's ability to bend the wrist back and straighten the fingers

- muscle weakness
- inability to extend one's fingers

verywell

Fig. 4. Radial nerve neuropathy. (*From* Chandra P, Kumar R, Mittal N. Recent developments in human gait research: Parameters, approaches, applications, machine learning techniques, datasets and challenges. The Artificial Intelligence Review. 2018;49(1):1-40.)

the findings, described previously. These help differentiate it from an injury at the spiral groove. It can occur following inappropriate use of crutches or tight clothing. In addition, the term, *Saturday night palsy*, is used, suggesting a prolonged period of arm immobilization with secondary nerve compression, such as after an extended period of draping the arm over a chair while inebriated. Symptoms may be immediate or delayed, occurring within days of the provoking event.

Another potential although controversial site of injury is at the elbow/proximal forearm, where the radial nerve forms the deep branch known as the posterior interosseous nerve (PIN). Here the PIN travels through the radial tunnel, a muscle-aponeurotic space extending from the lateral epicondyle to the distal margin of the supinator muscle.[8] Although PIN neuropathy can involve wrist and finger extensor weakness, radial tunnel syndrome often presents with pain at the lateral elbow, sometimes radiating down into the wrist, without associated weakness and with or without sensory complaints. Given the absence of objective signs, such as weakness, this often is misdiagnosed as refractory tennis elbow (lateral epicondylitis).[8]

In addition, isolated injury to smaller branches occasionally can be seen. For example, superficial radial nerve injury can occur above the wrist secondary to tight handcuffs or a tight watch, presenting with sensory changes and pain along the radial sensory distribution of the hand.

Peroneal Nerve Injury at the Fibular head

Fibular neuropathy, also known as peroneal neuropathy, is the most common entrapment neuropathy in the lower extremity, occurring at the level of the fibular head. The peroneal nerve fibers are derived from the L4-S1 nerve roots and travel through the sciatic nerve's fibular division over the posterior thigh before separating into the peroneal nerve. As the peroneal nerve wraps superficially around the fibular head at the lateral side of the knee, it is predisposed to compression, as shown in **Fig. 5.**

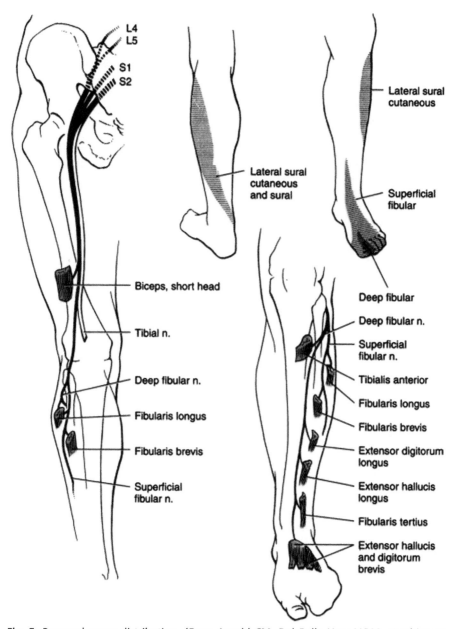

Fig. 5. Peroneal nerve distribution. (*From* Arnold CM, Dal Bello-Haas V.P.M., Farthing JP, et al. Falls and wrist fracture: Relationship to women's functional status after age 50. *Canadian Journal on Aging.* 2016;35(3):361-371.)

Clinically, peroneal nerve compression at the fibular head often presents as a foot drop and sensory changes at the dorsum of the foot. Neurologic examination may demonstrate weakness in foot dorsiflexion, eversion, and toe extension as well as sensory abnormalities in the distribution of the deep and superficial peroneal nerve fibers. The patient may complain of tripping over the affected foot or dragging it on the ground when walking. Presentation often is painless although burning, electrical pain, or skin sensitivity in the peroneal distribution may be seen. Habitual leg crossing is a common cause of this condition. Other causes include ganglion cyst in the popliteal fossa and direct nerve trauma or it can be secondary to local soft tissue swelling. Tapping of the nerve at the fibular head may result in tingling and electrical type pain down the leg and is suggestive of this condition (Tinel sign for the peroneal nerve). This presentation often can resemble sciatic neuropathy or L5 radiculopathy; therefore, additional testing, such as EMG/NCS and magnetic resonance imaging (MRI), can be helpful in making the final diagnosis. The differentiating factors are described in **Table 2**.

Peroneal neuropathy initially often is managed conservatively. The clinician should counsel the patient on avoiding putting pressure the nerve at the fibular head, including not crossing the legs when sitting and placing a pillow under the knee when sleeping on the affected side. Daily stretching of the ankle also is recommended for patients with foot drop to help in preventing contracture.

If weakness is present in toe extension only, sturdy footwear can help with walking.[9] If ankle dorsiflexion weakness is present, an ankle-foot orthosis brace can help with foot drop when walking to prevent tripping over the foot. Prolonged ankle immobilization should be avoided, however, to prevent muscle atrophy and contracture formation. Physical therapy also is important in helping with building muscle strength and gait and balance training. In refractory cases, surgical decompression may be considered.

Table 2
Differentiating factors in the cases of suspected sciatic neuropathy

	Deep Peroneal Nerve	Common Peroneal Nerve	Sciatic Nerve	Lumbosacral Plexus	L5
Weakness of foot dorsiflexion	X	X	X	X	X
Weakness of foot eversion		X	X	X	X
Weakness of foot inversion			X	X	X
Weakness of knee flexion			X	X	X
Weakness of glutei				X	X
Decreased ankle tendon reflex			X[a]	X[a]	X[a]
Sensory loss in webspace great toe	X	X	X	X	X
Sensory loss in dorsum of foot		X	X	X	X
Sensory loss in lateral calf		X	X	X	X
Sensory loss in lateral knee			X	X	X
Sensory loss in sole foot			X[a]	X[a]	X[a]
Sensory loss in posterior thigh				X[a]	X[a]
Tinel sign at fibular neck	X	X			
Hip and thigh pain			X	X	X
Back pain					X
Positive straight leg raise test					X

Abbreviation: X, may be present.
[a] May be present if lesion involves SI fibers as well.
From Naeem J, Nur AH, Islam MA, Amelia WA, Bijak M. Mechanomyography-based muscle fatigue detection during electrically elicited cycling in patients with spinal cord injury. *Medical and Biological Engineering and Computing.* 2019;57(6):1199-1211.

Sciatic Compression Neuropathy

The sciatic is the longest nerve in human body and injury can occur at multiple locations along its course. It arises from the lumbosacral plexus within the pelvis and travels under the gluteal compartment and down the posterior thigh, where it is composed of 2 distinct trunks, the common peroneal division, which sits laterally, and the tibial division, which sits medially. Within the posterior thigh, it separates into the distinct common peroneal and tibial nerves.

Within the pelvis, sciatic neuropathy can occur due to surgical manipulation, vaginal birth trauma, pelvic neoplasms, and endometriosis among others. Because the nerve and the hip joint have a close anatomic relationship, sciatic neuropathy can occur as a result of hip dislocation or iatrogenic injury during hip arthroplasty.

At the level of the gluteal compartment, injury can occur due to intramuscular injection. The sciatic nerve travels in the middle of the gluteal compartment below the piriformis. As a result, sciatic neuropathy is a well-recognized complication of gluteal intramuscular injection.[10] If gluteal injection is necessary, it should be done only in the upper-outer quadrant to avoid sciatic injury. Injury can range from mild (involving only pain or transient sensory changes down the leg) to severe (involving weakness in sciatic-innervated muscles of the leg).

Another potential and controversial cause of sciatic neuropathy is piriformis syndrome. This condition is felt to occur as result of piriformis spasm, trauma, or hypertrophy resulting in focal sciatic compression as the nerve travels through this muscle.[11]

Sciatic neuropathy often is present with both tibial and peroneal muscle weakness and sensory loss as well as absent ankle reflex on the affected side. Muscle weakness classically involves foot dorsiflexion, plantarflexion, eversion, and inversion as well as toe flexors and extensors. More proximal muscles, including the knee flexors (also known as hamstring muscles), also may be affected. A sciatic neuropathy, however, also can have a strong clinical resemblance to a peroneal neuropathy. This is due to the lateral positioning of peroneal fibers within the sciatic nerve, resulting in higher susceptibility to stretch and compression injury. In this setting, the patient may present with weakness in dorsiflexion, eversion and toe extension only, and EMG/NCS is important to distinguish between the 2 conditions. In addition, the differential diagnosis may also include L5-S1 radiculopathy and lumbosacral plexopathy. Detailed history and clinical examination are crucial in determining the correct diagnosis. **Table 2** lists the clinically differentiating factors between the different conditions.

DIAGNOSTIC WORK-UP FOR MONONEUROPATHIES

When evaluating for a potential entrapment mononeuropathy, a detailed history and physical examination are the first and most crucial steps in localizing the lesion. The clinician should elicit any history of associated trauma or other inciting event leading to the presentation, along with any history of similar events in the past. Duration and progression of symptoms are important as well. Physical examination should involve a detailed examination of muscle strength and sensory function in the multiple nerve and nerve root distributions of all 4 limbs. Deep tendon reflexes should be evaluated both to help identify the affected nerve as well as rule out an upper motor neuron lesion, such as stroke. Although rare, upper motor neuron lesions, such as acute ischemic stroke, can mimic an entrapment neuropathy.[12] Often EMG/NCS is helpful to confirm the site of the lesion as well as determine the degree of nerve injury and prognosis. In addition, electrodiagnostic testing can be helpful in ruling out alternative causes in the peripheral nervous system, such as plexopathy, radiculopathy, and motor neuron disease. If cervical or lumbar radiculopathy is suspected, then dedicated imaging of the spinal segment is important as well. Neuromuscular ultrasound, although not used as commonly, can be helpful in visualizing the affected nerve and the surrounding structures. Focal nerve edema can be identified by increased cross-sectional area, change in echogenicity, and altered fascicular pattern.[13] Although helpful in confirming the diagnosis, this imaging modality is inferior to EMG/NCS when it comes to determining the severity of injury and prognosis. In cases of moderate to severe or refractory entrapment neuropathy, MRI of the associated area can be considered to look for compressive mass lesions, such as cysts and tumors.

In the setting of trauma, a prompt evaluation by orthopedics is important. Peripheral nerve reconstruction and decompression following severe injury or transection in the acute, posttraumatic setting may be warranted.

If the presentation is atypical and concerning for more of a systemic or multifocal process, the patient should receive a comprehensive neurologic evaluation. Bloodwork can be done to look for additional causes of neuropathy, including complete blood cell count, basic metabolic panel, fasting blood glucose, thyroid function tests, vitamin B_{12}, and paraproteinemia work-up, including serum protein electrophoresis and immunofixation. Other tests, such as Lyme serology, human immunodeficiency virus serology, vitamin D, vitamin B_6, antinuclear antibody, and additional inflammatory studies, can be considered. If a patient has a history of multiple compressive neuropathies and/or strong family history of compressive neuropathies, a hereditary neuropathy syndrome may be considered, such as hereditary neuropathy with liability to pressure palsy or familial amyloidosis.

MANAGEMENT OPTIONS

In the setting of nontraumatic, mild to moderate entrapment neuropathies, management often initially is conservative. This involves stabilizing the associated joint and avoiding triggering activities, although prolonged immobilization is not recommended. Patient education, therefore, is crucial. Neuropathic pain medication can be given to alleviate positive symptoms, such as burning and electrical pain, tingling, and skin sensitivity. This may include antiepileptic agents, such as gabapentin or pregabalin, which are used most commonly. Additional antiepileptic agents, however, including lamotrigine, carbamazepine, and oxcarbazepine, also have been used, although efficacy has not been well established.[14] Antidepressants are an alternative category of neuropathic agents that often are used. These include duloxetine, venlafaxine, amitriptyline, and nortriptyline. Additional therapies include nonsteroidal anti-inflammatory drugs, and acetaminophen can be helpful in treating both neuropathic and nociceptive pain. If weakness in the affected muscles is present, physical therapy and occupational therapy are important as well. In more severe, refractory cases, more invasive techniques, including injections and surgical decompression, can be performed. In the setting of a compressive lesion, such as a tumor or ganglion cyst, surgical options should be considered early.

SUMMARY

Entrapment neuropathies are common conditions seen by clinicians in a wide range of specialties. These injuries often are due to external compression or stretch of the affected nerve; therefore, patient education, activity, and position modifications are the mainstays of treatment. Often, conservative management is the initial treatment preferred. When conservative management fails or in cases of open injuries or significant associated weakness, however, surgical options are available and effective.

CLINICS CARE POINTS

- Entrapment neuropathies often present slowly, although they can present acutely, especially in the case of trauma.

- Positive Tinel sign on physical examination occurs when tapping over the affected nerve triggers a patient's symptoms. This examination finding can help support a diagnosis of compression neuropathy at multiple entrapment sites.

- Phalen maneuver, a physical examination maneuver in the diagnosis of CTS, involves having the patient forcibly flex the wrists for up to 1 minute and monitoring for symptom exacerbation.

- Weakness and atrophy of affected muscles on examination should warrant a surgical evaluation.

- Conservative therapy may involve splinting, associated joint immobilization, and avoiding triggering activities.

- Saturday night palsy refers to radial nerve compression secondary to prolonged period of arm immobilization.

- Due to lateral positioning of peroneal fibers in the sciatic nerve, compressive sciatic neuropathy clinically may resemble a peroneal neuropathy, and EMG/NCS is important to distinguish between the 2 conditions.

- Differential diagnosis of a compressive mononeuropathy may include radiculopathy, plexopathy, and an upper motor neuron lesion. Careful clinical examination is crucial, and EMG/NCS can be helpful in further localizing the lesion.

- Neuropathic pain medications that can help with the treatment of positive symptoms include antidepressants and antiepileptics. These agents are not effective in treating the negative symptoms of neuropathy.

DISCLOSURE

The authors have nothing to disclose.

REFERENCES

1. Dy CJ, Mackinnon SE. Ulnar neuropathy: evaluation and management. Curr Rev Musculoskelet Med 2016;9(2):178–84.
2. Aroori S, Spence RA. Carpal tunnel syndrome. Ulster Med J 2008;77(1):6–17.
3. Eisenbud L, Ejadi S, Mar N. Development of carpal tunnel syndrome in association with checkpoint inhibitors. J Oncol Pharm Pract 2020. https://doi.org/10.1177/1078155220950430. 1078155220950430.
4. Quan D, Bird S. Nerve conduction studies and electromyography in the evaluation of peripheral nerve injuries. UPOJ 1999;12:45–51.
5. Andrews K, Rowland A, Pranjal A, et al. Cubital tunnel syndrome: anatomy, clinical presentation, and management. J Orthop 2018;15(3):832–6.
6. Aleksenko D, Varacallo M. Guyon canal syndrome. In: StatPearls. Treasure Island (FL): StatPearls Publishing; 2020. Available at: https://www.ncbi.nlm.nih.gov/books/NBK431063/.
7. Shah CM, Calfee RP, Gelberman RH, et al. Outcomes of rigid night splinting and activity modification in the treatment of cubital tunnel syndrome. J Hand Surg Am 2013;38(6):1125–30.e1.

8. Caetano EB, Vieira LA, Sabongi Neto JJ, et al. Anatomical study of radial tunnel and its clinical implications in compressive syndromes. Rev Bras Ortop (Sao Paulo) 2020;55(1):27–32.

9. Chandra P, Kumar R, Mittal N. Recent developments in human gait research: Parameters, approaches, applications, machine learning techniques, datasets and challenges. Artif Intelligence Rev 2018;49(1):1–40.

10. Mishra P, Stringer MD. Sciatic nerve injury from intramuscular injection: a persistent and global problem. Int J Clin Pract 2010;64(11):1573–9.

11. Hicks BL, Lam JC, Varacallo M. Piriformis syndrome. In: StatPearls. Treasure Island (FL): StatPearls Publishing; 2020. Available at: https://www.ncbi.nlm.nih.gov/books/NBK448172/.

12. Tahir H, Daruwalla V, Meisel J, et al. Pseudoradial nerve palsy caused by acute ischemic stroke. J Investig Med High Impact Case Rep 2016;4(3). 2324709616658310.

13. Choi SJ, Ahn JH, Ryu DS, et al. Ultrasonography for nerve compression syndromes of the upper extremity. Ultrasonography 2015;34(4):275–91.

14. Wiffen PJ, Derry S, Moore RA, et al. Antiepileptic drugs for neuropathic pain and fibromyalgia - an overview of Cochrane reviews. Cochrane Database Syst Rev 2013;(11):CD010567. Accessed 02 December 2020.

Diabetes and Peripheral Nerve Disease

Lindsay A. Zilliox, MD, MS

KEYWORDS

- Diabetes • Neuropathy • Diabetic neuropathy • Impaired glucose tolerance
- Metabolic syndrome • Autonomic neuropathy • Diabetic amyotrophy

KEY POINTS

- Typical distal symmetric polyneuropathy presents with numbness or paresthesias of the feet that is symmetric with minimal weakness and progresses gradually in a length-dependent fashion.
- Patients with an idiopathic painful peripheral neuropathy should be screened for prediabetes.
- Neuropathy in type 1 diabetes is closely linked to hyperglycemia. However, in type 2 diabetes, the risk of neuropathy is associated with hyperglycemia, as well as additional factors including: hypertension, hyperlipidemia, obesity, and tobacco use.
- Complications of diabetic neuropathy include foot ulcerations and amputations, increased risk of falls, and difficult-to-control neuropathic pain, and patients with diabetic cardiovascular autonomic neuropathy have an increased risk of mortality.

INTRODUCTION

There is a global epidemic of diabetes and prediabetes with their associated complications. The International Diabetes Federation estimates that 463 million people in the world have diabetes, and the proportion of people with type 2 diabetes (T2DM) continues to increase. An equally alarming, but often underappreciated fact is that an additional 374 million people are estimated to have prediabetes.[1] Among those with diabetes, approximately 50% will develop neuropathy, which is the most common and costly complication of diabetes. A growing body of literature recognized prediabetes and the metabolic syndrome as risk factors for neuropathy. It is estimated that 10% of patients with prediabetes have neuropathy. Diabetic neuropathy encompasses a group of clinical syndromes caused by damage to peripheral and autonomic nerves. The most common form of diabetic neuropathy is a "typical" distal symmetric polyneuropathy, but other neuropathies also occur and are referred to in this article as "atypical diabetic neuropathy."

Department of Neurology, University of Maryland School of Medicine & Maryland VA Healthcare System, 3S-130, 110 South Paca Street, Baltimore, MD 21201-1595, USA
E-mail address: lzilliox@som.umaryland.edu

Clin Geriatr Med 37 (2021) 253–267
https://doi.org/10.1016/j.cger.2020.12.001
0749-0690/21/Published by Elsevier Inc.
geriatric.theclinics.com

Diabetic neuropathy is a major public health concern and a leading source of morbidity and mortality as well as health care resources. Diabetic autonomic neuropathy is associated with an increased risk of cardiovascular mortality,[2] and diabetic peripheral neuropathy is associated with foot ulceration, leading to lower-limb amputation and increased risk of death.[3] In addition, more than 20% of patients with diabetic neuropathy have severe pain that adversely impacts their daily activities, sleep, and overall quality of life. Patients with severe neuropathic pain are often difficult to treat and incur greater health care costs than those without pain. Another complication of diabetic neuropathy, which stems from the loss of position sense and distal weakness, is falls. Currently, there are no known disease-modifying therapies for diabetic neuropathy, so early diagnosis and prevention or delay of long-term complications is of paramount importance.

DIABETES, PREDIABETES, AND NEUROPATHY

Neuropathy can occur in all forms of diabetes, although T2DM accounts for most cases of diabetic neuropathy because of its ever-increasing prevalence. Although neuropathy was traditionally thought to be a late complication of diabetes, it is increasingly recognized that it can occur at the earliest stages of glucose dysregulation, such as occurs with prediabetes and the metabolic syndrome. At the time of diagnosis of diabetes, nerve conduction studies are abnormal in 20% of patients, which indicates that neuropathy is already present.[4] There is also an epidemiologic association between impaired glucose tolerance and an increased risk of neuropathy. Up to 50% of patients with an idiopathic neuropathy have impaired glucose tolerance.[5] In addition, the prevalence of neuropathy in patients with both impaired fasting glucose and impaired glucose tolerance (23.9%) has been found to be close to those with known T2DM (22.0%).[6] These findings support the recommendation that in patients with an otherwise idiopathic neuropathy, screening for prediabetes and diabetes with a glycosylated hemoglobin (HbA$_{1c}$) and a 2-hour oral glucose tolerance test should be considered. Diagnostic criteria for diabetes and prediabetes are shown in **Table 1**.

TYPICAL DISTAL SYMMETRIC POLYNEUROPATHY

Typical distal symmetric polyneuropathy, which is the most common type of diabetic neuropathy, is characterized by slowly progressive, symmetric sensory loss that is often accompanied by pain. There is a gradual onset of distal paresthesias, which may or may not be painful, or numbness that is eventually followed by motor weakness. The "stocking-glove" or "dying back" pattern of sensory abnormalities is characteristic of a metabolic neuropathy with preferential damage to the longest axons first. Patients may complain of so-called negative symptoms, including numbness, which they may or may not be aware of, or positive symptoms, such as prickling,

Table 1 Diagnostic criteria for diabetes and prediabetes			
	Normal	Prediabetes	Diabetes
Fasting plasma glucose, mg/dL	<100	100–125	≥126
2-h oral glucose tolerance test, mg/dL	<140	140–199	≥200
Glycosylated hemoglobin, %	<5.7	5.7-6.4	≥6.5
Random plasma glucose, mg/dL			≥200

burning, or aching paresthesias. Typically, sensory symptoms and pain are worse at rest or at night.

The neuropathy that is characteristically seen in prediabetes and early diabetes affects unmyelinated, small-diameter nerve fibers. These nerve fibers carry pain, temperature sensation, and peripheral autonomic function. Patients with a small-fiber neuropathy typically complain of burning neuropathic pain, and on examination, they have abnormalities on pinprick and temperature sensation testing (**Table 2**). The damaged peripheral autonomic fibers lead to alterations in sweating, and one can see skin changes with dryness, edema, or pallor of the distal lower extremities. Strength testing and deep tendon reflexes are preserved, and sensory testing to vibration and proprioception is normal. Nerve conduction studies may be normal with a small-fiber neuropathy.

As diabetes progresses, there is eventually involvement of large-diameter nerve fibers, and clinically there is impairment of vibratory sensation, proprioception, and reduced reflexes. Significant weakness is not common in early diabetic neuropathy, although there may be weakness of toe flexor or extensor muscles. Some patients with diabetic neuropathy are not aware of their sensory loss, and if undiagnosed, they can experience painless injuries. These individuals are especially prone to developing foot ulcerations and are at a higher risk of falls.

SCREENING AND DIAGNOSIS

Because of a current lack of disease-modifying treatments, the early diagnosis of diabetic neuropathy is essential for delaying or preventing the development of complications, such as ulcerations and amputations. Diabetic neuropathy likely begins with reversible physiologic abnormalities that then progress to irreversible axonal damage, and the early diagnosis of neuropathy will likely be an essential first step for any effective treatment. The American Diabetes Association (ADA) recommends screening for neuropathy in any patient with type 1 diabetes (T1DM) for more than 5 years and any patient with T2DM with subsequent annual screenings.[7] In addition, one should suspect neuropathy because of prediabetes in any patient with an idiopathic painful polyneuropathy. Prediabetes is found in 40% to 50% of patients with idiopathic polyneuropathy compared with 14% of the age-matched general population.[8]

Screening for diabetic neuropathy should include a careful history and clinical assessment of small-fiber function (sensation to temperature or pin prick) and large-fiber nerve

Table 2
Small-fiber versus large-fiber neuropathy

	Small-Fiber Neuropathy	Large-Fiber Neuropathy
Clinical Presentation	Pain Predominates	Imbalance, Weakness
Physical examination	• Reduced sensation to pinprick and temperature • Reduced distal sweating pattern with increased sweating more proximally, dry skin; feet are cool to the touch and may appear pale	• Reduced proprioception and vibratory sensation • Reduced deep tendon reflexes
Confirmatory testing	• Skin biopsy for measurement of intraepidermal nerve fiber density • Quantitative sudomotor axon reflex test	• Abnormalities on nerve conduction testing

function (sensation to vibration with a 128-Hz tuning fork, proprioception, light touch with 10-g monofilament, and deep tendon reflexes at the ankle) (**Box 1**). One should also consider potential alternative or additional causes of neuropathy as well (**Box 2**). Most patients with typical signs and symptoms of diabetic neuropathy do not require routine confirmatory testing for the diagnosis of typical distal symmetric polyneuropathy in diabetes. However, testing may be helpful if there are any atypical clinical features. Atypical features include significant asymmetry on examination, early weakness, and an acute onset or rapidly progressive course.

Confirmatory testing for neuropathy often entails electrodiagnostic testing, including nerve conduction studies that assess large-fiber function. Typical changes seen in diabetic neuropathy reflect axonal loss and include reduced amplitudes and mild decrease in conduction velocities. These changes are seen in a length-dependent fashion with abnormalities in the lower limbs first. An important caveat is that nerve conduction tests do not assess small-fiber function. Skin punch biopsies with measurement of intraepidermal nerve fiber density (IENFD) are sometimes used in the diagnosis of small-fiber neuropathy. Other confirmatory tests of small-fiber nerve damage include quantitative sensory thermal thresholds for reduced cooling detection thresholds or elevated heat thresholds and corneal confocal microscopy to measure nerve fiber length.

RISK FACTORS AND PATHOPHYSIOLOGY

It is well recognized that the prevalence of diabetic neuropathy increases with the duration and severity of hyperglycemia. However, other modifiable risk factors have also been identified. Hyperglycemia is the major driving factor of neuropathy in T1DM, but hypertension, serum lipids and triglycerides, body mass index, and smoking have been found to be independent risk factors.[9] In T2DM, hyperglycemia plays a smaller role in the development and progression of neuropathy, whereas metabolic

---

Box 1
Characteristic history and physical examination in typical diabetic sensorimotor peripheral neuropathy

History
- Symptoms start in the toes with slow progression more proximally
- Early symptoms include numbness or tingling sensations
- Symptoms are worse at night
- Imbalance when walking at night or on uneven surfaces

Physical examination
- Pinprick and temperature sensation reduced at the distal lower extremities
- Vibration and proprioception reduced at the great toe
- Loss of ankle reflexes
- Weakness of toe flexion/extension or ankle dorsiflexion/plantarflexion
- Romberg test of proprioception
- Assess normal and tandem gait

Red flags
- Significant weakness early in the disease course
- Significant asymmetry of signs or symptoms
- Rapidly progressive course
- Prominent autonomic symptoms early in the disease course (lightheadedness, constipation, urinary retention)
- Family history of neuropathy
- History of heavy alcohol use

| Box 2 |
| Potential alternative causes of diabetic neuropathy |

- Vitamin B12 deficiency
- Alcohol use
- Paraproteinemia (serum protein electrophoresis and immunofixation)
- Chronic kidney disease
- Chemotherapy
- Hereditary neuropathy
- Chronic inflammatory demyelinating polyneuropathy

syndrome, especially the components of obesity and hyperlipidemia, and tobacco use are significant independent risk factors for diabetic neuropathy.[10–13] Supporting the independent role of the metabolic syndrome on the development of diabetic neuropathy is the finding that, regardless of glucose control, patients with an idiopathic neuropathy are more likely than the general population to have features of the metabolic syndrome, including obesity, hypertension, and dyslipidemia.[14]

PATHOPHYSIOLOGY

As previously mentioned, diabetic neuropathies preferentially affect sensory neurons. In particular, unmyelinated small-diameter sensory axons are especially susceptible to damage, and the "dying back," length-dependent pattern of progression reflects damage to the longest sensory axons first. The underlying pathogenesis of diabetic neuropathy remains incompletely understood, and a detailed review is outside the scope of this article. However, it is clear that persistent hyperglycemia along with additional metabolic derangements related to impaired insulin signaling, hyperlipidemia, and adiposity trigger changes in multiple biochemical pathways (polyol and hexosamine pathways and the formation of reactive oxygen species and advanced glycation end products) that result in damage to mitochondria and an overall increase in oxidative stress and inflammation that ultimately results in nerve injury. In addition, diabetes is associated with a microangiopathy, and nerve biopsy samples from patients with diabetic neuropathy demonstrate thickened endoneurial blood vessel walls.[15] The ultimate result is peripheral nerve ischemia owing to endothelial injury and microvascular dysfunction. To compound the ongoing nerve damage, peripheral nerve repair is also impaired in diabetes.[16]

PREVENTION OF DIABETIC NEUROPATHY
Glucose Control

Tight glucose control has been shown to reduce the incidence of neuropathy in patients with T1DM, but there is no convincing evidence in T2DM for more than a modest effect on neuropathy outcomes.[17,18] Glucose control probably plays an important part of neuropathy prevention in T2DM, but it is not sufficient alone, and other risk factors likely play an important role in neuropathy risk. This fact reflects the differences in the underlying pathophysiology of neuropathy in T1DM and T2DM.

The Diabetes Control and Complications Trial showed that more intensive glucose control prevented the onset and progression of both peripheral and cardiac autonomic neuropathy in patients with T1DM. In fact, there was a 64% reduced risk of peripheral neuropathy and a 45% reduced risk of cardiac autonomic neuropathy over 5 years.[19]

Furthermore, once the intervention was over and both groups of participants were instructed on strict glucose control, the prevalence and incidence of neuropathy remained significantly lower in the former intensive therapy group compared with the former conventional therapy group for an additional 14 years, despite similar glucose control in both groups.[20] This persistent effect of early intensive glucose control has been termed "metabolic memory" and underscores the importance of the early diagnosis and treatment of diabetic neuropathy.

Although strict glucose control alone is not enough to convincingly prevent or slow the progression of neuropathy, the choice of diabetes medication might have an impact. A study of the effect of insulin-sensitizing (metformin, thiazolidinediones, or both) versus insulin-providing treatments (sulfonylureas/meglitinides, insulin, or both) on cardiovascular outcomes in T2DM found that the type of glucose-lowering agent used to obtain normoglycemia may make a difference in preventing the development of neuropathy in patients with T2DM. After adjusting for HbA$_{1c}$, the insulin-sensitizing treatments were associated with a reduced development of peripheral neuropathy in T2DM compared with insulin-providing treatments.[21] The reduced incidence of peripheral neuropathy in T2DM patients treated with insulin sensitizing treatments suggests that medications that are used to treat hyperglycemia may also have additional, independent effects on other pathways, such as chronic inflammation, lipid metabolism, body weight, or oxidative stress, that are involved in the development of neuropathy in T2DM.

Lifestyle Interventions

Lifestyle interventions that include exercise and dietary changes are an attractive treatment for diabetic neuropathy because they target several of the pathways and risk factors that are implicated in the development of diabetic neuropathy. Although the Diabetes Prevention Program (DPP) demonstrated that physical activity and dietary changes were effective in reducing the incidence of T2DM in people with impaired glucose tolerance, there was no difference in microvascular outcomes, including peripheral neuropathy.[22] However, when examining the cohort of patients who developed T2DM, the individuals who were in the lifestyle intervention group did have a lower prevalence of neuropathy compared with those who received standard care.[23] The same lifestyle intervention that was used in the DPP was used in a year-long natural history study of patients with impaired glucose tolerance and neuropathy. Individuals who lost weight and/or increased their physical activity were found to have significantly increased IENFD at the proximal thigh. This improvement in a pathologic measure of small-fiber neuropathy was significantly correlated with the clinically relevant outcome measurement of decreased neuropathic pain.[24], which suggests that aggressive treatment of prediabetes with a lifestyle intervention might improve clinically relevant measures of neuropathy and highlights the importance of action during the earliest stages of impaired glucose regulation.

Studies of patients with metabolic syndrome or T2DM and no signs or symptoms of neuropathy at baseline found that those assigned to a weekly exercise program had a significantly increased distal leg IENFD[25] and cutaneous nerve regenerative capacity[26] compared with those who received health counseling. These results suggest that not only does exercise have the potential to prevent nerve injury but also it may promote nerve regeneration. Several small uncontrolled trials have shown that exercise has a possible role in the prevention of diabetic neuropathy. Taken together, an exercise program is an important part of the treatment plan for all patients with diabetes. The ADA recommends a goal of 150 minutes of at least moderate-intensity aerobic activity and 2 to 3 sessions of resistance training each week.[27]

TREATMENT OF DIABETIC NEUROPATHY
Disease-Modifying Treatment

In general, patients with diabetic neuropathy are encouraged to not only optimize their glycemic control but also aggressively treat their lipids and blood pressure along with lifestyle modifications to increase their amount of exercise, lose weight, and stop smoking. Although there are no treatments that have been proven to reverse diabetic neuropathy, there are promising data to suggest that lifestyle interventions may be able to improve measures of diabetic neuropathy. However, it remains unknown exactly what the optimal exercise routine entails, what dietary changes should be, and if lifestyle interventions will be effective for all patients with diabetic neuropathy or just those at the early stages of the disease.

There is some evidence that lifestyle interventions may be effective not only in the prevention of but also as a treatment for established diabetic neuropathy. A pilot study of patients with T2DM and neuropathy found an improvement in neuropathic symptoms and the intraepidermal nerve fiber branching from skin biopsies at the proximal thigh in patients who participated in 10 weeks of aerobic and strength training exercise.[28] This study was a pilot study and requires additional testing, but the results demonstrated evidence of nerve regeneration and were consistent with findings of longer studies.[24]

There have been many pharmaceutical agents that have been studied in diabetic neuropathy. Many treatments, however, have not been successful in clinical trials either because of poor efficacy or intolerable side effects. The lack of efficacy from drug trials may be due to targeting only individual pathways involved in the pathogenesis of diabetic neuropathy, which may not be enough to combat the cascade of changes in multiple interconnected pathways that ultimately result in axonal damage. Therefore, the major goal of treatment remains treatment of modifiable risk factors.

Symptomatic Treatment

The goal of disease-modifying treatments is to reverse damage to peripheral nerves in diabetic neuropathy. However, at the present time, treatment options are limited, and the focus of most clinic appointments with patients centers on symptomatic treatment, including neuropathic pain control and prevention of complications such as foot ulcers and falls. All patients with diabetic neuropathy should be educated on proper foot care. Proper foot care should include daily inspection of the feet and skin care to avoid dry or cracking skin, fissures, or callus formation. In addition, patients should be educated on the gait instability and risk of falls associated with diabetic neuropathy because of loss of position sense, foot pain, orthostatic hypotension, age-related functional impairments, and medication side effects. Exercise programs, including physical and occupations therapy, may be required as well as home safety evaluations and the need for equipment, such as handlebars and night lights.

Approximately one-quarter of patients with diabetic neuropathy have painful symptoms, and this is often the reason that patients seek care. It is important to address pain at each visit with patients because not only can pain limit function but also it adversely affects quality of life. Treatment of neuropathic pain is covered by Elizabeth J. Pedowitz and colleagues' article, "Management of Neuropathic Pain in the Geriatric Population," in this issue and will not be extensively covered here. The initial choice of pharmacologic therapy for painful diabetic neuropathy includes antidepressants (tricyclic antidepressants or serotonin-norepinephrine reuptake inhibitors) and gabapentinoids. The Food and Drug Administration has approved duloxetine, pregabalin, and the capsaicin patch for the treatment of painful diabetic neuropathy, and opioids are typically avoided in the treatment of painful diabetic neuropathy. There are published guidelines for the treatment of painful diabetic neuropathy.[29]

Dietary supplements have also been another area of interest in the treatment of diabetic neuropathy. Alpha-lipoic acid is an antioxidant that has been studied in several clinical trials and has been shown to improve measures and symptoms of neuropathy at a dose of 600 mg daily.[30,31] There is also preliminary evidence that dietary supplementation with seal oil omega-3 polyunsaturated fatty acids may improve measures of small-fiber neuropathy in patients with T1DM and neuropathy,[32] but confirmatory studies are needed.

DIABETIC AUTONOMIC NEUROPATHY

Diabetic autonomic neuropathy is a common manifestation of diabetic neuropathy, but it is often underrecognized. However, it is important to diagnose because of the association of cardiac autonomic neuropathy with an increased mortality risk. Part of the reason diabetic autonomic neuropathy requires a high index of suspicion is because of its slow onset with multiorgan involvement and vague symptoms. There are validated questionnaires, such as the Survey of Autonomic Symptoms,[33] that can increase the diagnostic sensitivity, but symptoms alone are not sufficient to make a diagnosis of diabetic autonomic neuropathy. Testing modalities are outlined in **Table 3**, and in general, abnormalities in tests of both the sympathetic and the parasympathetic pathways are required for a definite diagnosis. Reports of the prevalence of diabetic autonomic neuropathy range widely because of the lack of standardized measures for diagnosis. Diabetic autonomic neuropathy is associated with age, poor glucose control, vascular risk factors, and the coexistence of diabetic peripheral neuropathy.

Cardiovascular Autonomic Neuropathy

One of the earliest signs of cardiovascular autonomic neuropathy is a resting tachycardia, and one of the most sensitive tests is the heart rate response to deep breathing (expiration:inspiration ratio). Resting tachycardia and decreased heart rate variability in response to deep breathing is due to early involvement of the vagus nerve, one of the longest nerves, in diabetes. Damage to the vagus nerve results in a decrease in vagal tone and a relative predominance of the sympathetic nervous system. As the cardiovascular autonomic neuropathy progresses, the heart rate slows, and eventually, there is a fixed heart rate and lack of variability because of cardiac denervation. Other clinical manifestations of cardiovascular autonomic neuropathy include exercise intolerance, orthostatic hypotension, syncope, intraoperative cardiovascular instability, silent myocardial infarction and ischemia, and ultimately, increased cardiac and all-cause mortality. Orthostatic hypotension is the symptom that causes the highest level of morbidity in patients with cardiovascular autonomic neuropathy. The first step in the treatment of patients with orthostatic hypotension should be to remove any medication that can cause or exacerbate orthostatic hypotension. In addition, one should ensure adequate volume repletion and educate patients on physical activity and the use of compression garments before starting a trial of low-dose fludrocortisone or midodrine. A major complication in the treatment of orthostatic hypotension is the supine hypertension that is often seen in patients with diabetic cardiovascular autonomic neuropathy, which can be exacerbated by the use of medications to treat orthostatic hypotension. In these patients, timing of medications is very important, and the use of a short-acting antihypertensive may be needed before bedtime.

The association between cardiovascular autonomic neuropathy in diabetes and mortality is high. A meta-analysis of patients with diabetes found that those without

Table 3
Symptoms and testing modalities for diabetic autonomic neuropathy

Category of Diabetic Autonomic Neuropathy	Symptoms	Potential Offending Medications	Diagnostic Tests
Cardiovascular	Orthostatic hypotension Arrhythmia Reduced exercise tolerance	Antidepressants, antihypertensives, alpha-1 blockers, dopaminergic agents	Heart rate response to deep breathing Valsalva response Head up tilt table
Gastrointestinal	Nausea and vomiting Early satiety Constipation/diarrhea Gastroesophageal reflux disease Poor glycemic control	Opioids, clonidine, tricyclic antidepressants, calcium channel blockers, dopaminergic agents, anticholinergics, glucagonlike peptide 1 agonists, phenothiazine, cyclosporine	Gastric-emptying study Colonoscopy
Urogenital	Neurogenic bladder Frequent urinary tract infections Erectile dysfunction Retrograde ejaculation Reduced vaginal lubrication	Anticholinergics, tricyclic antidepressants, calcium channel blockers, alpha-1 blockers, and alpha-1 agonists	Postvoid residual Nocturnal penile plethysmography
Peripheral	Distal anhidrosis Proximal hyperhidrosis Heat intolerance Dry skin	Drugs causing hyperhidrosis: Anticholinesterases, antidepressants, opioids, muscarinic agonists Drugs causing hypohidrosis: Anticholinergics, antidepressants, antiepileptics, antihistamines, clonidine, antimuscarinics, muscle relaxants, opioids	Quantitative sudomotor axon reflex test Sympathetic skin response Thermoregulatory sweat testing

autonomic neuropathy had a mortality of 5% over 5.5 years, but the mortality increased to 27% in patients with cardiac autonomic neuropathy.[2] In patients with T1DM, there is evidence that intensive glucose control can reduce the incidence of cardiac autonomic neuropathy by 53%.[34] However, similar to peripheral neuropathy, strict glucose control has much less of an effect in T2DM. In patients with T2DM, treatment of cardiovascular autonomic neuropathy consists of not only glucose control but also modification of other vascular risk factors and smoking cessation. At this time, there is no specific disease-modifying treatment for cardiac autonomic neuropathy, and symptomatic treatments do not affect mortality.

Gastrointestinal Autonomic Neuropathy

Gastrointestinal autonomic dysfunction commonly leads to gastroparesis, which is defined as retained food in the stomach 8 hours after a meal. Gastroparesis is associated with symptoms including nausea, vomiting, bloating, and early satiety. Importantly, the slowed intestinal absorption of glucose because of gastroparesis can complicate postprandial insulin administration and lead to hypoglycemia. The resulting variability in glucose levels can lead to difficult-to-control diabetes. Another relatively common manifestation of gastrointestinal autonomic neuropathy is esophageal dysfunction that can result in dysphagia and gastroesophageal reflux disease. Chronic constipation or diarrhea can also occur in patients with diabetic autonomic neuropathy. These conditions are common and require a high degree of suspicion to diagnose as being due to diabetic gastrointestinal autonomic neuropathy.

Urogenital Autonomic Neuropathy

Urogenital autonomic dysfunction can lead to bladder and sexual dysfunction. Symptoms of bladder dysfunction include both urinary hesitancy and retention or urinary urgency and incontinence. Initially, there is an impairment in the sensation of bladder fullness, and as the neuropathy progresses, there is dysfunction of the detrusor that can eventually lead to urinary retention. All of these factors increase the risk of recurrent urinary tract infections.

Symptoms of sexual dysfunction owing to diabetic autonomic neuropathy include impotence, decreased libido, erectile dysfunction, or abnormal ejaculation in men or painful intercourse and reduced libido in women. Erectile dysfunction in particular is highly prevalent in men with diabetes and is the most common symptom in men with diabetic autonomic neuropathy. In addition, erectile dysfunction is a marker of cardiovascular disease in diabetes and is an independent risk factor for cardiovascular events.[35] Bladder and sexual dysfunction are both also frequently due to medication side effects, and an initial step in their evaluation is removing any potentially offending medications (see **Table 3**).

Peripheral Autonomic Neuropathy

Diabetic autonomic neuropathy affects the peripheral sympathetic cholinergic nerves in a length-dependent fashion similar to typical distal symmetric polyneuropathy. Sudomotor autonomic dysfunction mainly affects sweating and thermoregulation and manifests with dry skin, edema, pallor, and decreased sweating distally with compensatory proximal hyperhidrosis. Patients frequently complain of hyperhidrosis, but it is important to recognize that this is to compensate for hypohidrosis in another area, and treatment can potentially lead to hyperthermia. Because peripheral autonomic neuropathy is due to dysfunction of small unmyelinated nerve fibers, it is frequently the earliest clinical manifestation of diabetic neuropathy and can occur when patients are prediabetic. In the later stages, peripheral autonomic neuropathy may be a contributing factor to the development of foot ulceration and ultimately amputation.

"ATYPICAL DIABETIC NEUROPATHIES"
Polyradiculopathies and Diabetic Radiculoplexus Neuropathy

Polyradiculopathies, or damage to nerve roots, usually occur in diabetes at thoracic or high lumbar levels and can extend over time to adjacent levels. Patients are typically older with an existing peripheral neuropathy and have weakness and atrophy in the distribution of one or more nerve roots. One common type of diabetic polyradiculopathy is diabetic lumbosacral radiculoplexus neuropathy, which is commonly referred to as diabetic amyotrophy. It is relatively uncommon and typically presents subacutely over weeks or months with asymmetrical lower-extremity pain followed by weakness and muscle atrophy that can spread to the contralateral limb over time. The typical patient is a man over 50 years old with well-controlled T2DM. The syndrome is often heralded by unexplained weight loss (median of 30 pounds). Severe and lancinating pain precedes the weakness and typically starts off unilaterally in the low back, hip, or thigh. Days to weeks later, the affected leg develops significant weakness and atrophy. The proximal hip and knee muscles are affected most commonly, but distal leg weakness with foot drop can also occur. The illness is generally monophasic but can progress over the course of many months (median 5 months) before reaching its nadir. Recovery can take up to 24 months, and although most patients do improve, there is frequently incomplete recovery. Most patients will eventually require assistance with ambulation, with foot drop being a common permanent deficit.

In diabetic lumbosacral radiculoplexus neuropathy, there is involvement of not only multiple lumbosacral nerve roots but also the lumbosacral plexus and peripheral nerves. The extent of involvement can be demonstrated on electrodiagnostic testing to confirm the diagnosis. The underlying pathophysiology is not directly related to hyperglycemia and is most likely due to ischemic injury. Despite some success of immunosuppressive treatment with intravenous methylprednisolone on pain control,[36] there is no proven effective treatment, and management remains supportive.

Focal Neuropathies

Compressive neuropathies, including median mononeuropathy at the wrist (carpal tunnel syndrome), ulnar mononeuropathy at the elbow (cubital tunnel syndrome), and peroneal mononeuropathy at the fibular head, are more common in patients with diabetes than the general population. The clinical presentation is the same, but the diagnosis can be more challenging because of the coexisting peripheral neuropathy.

Cranial mononeuropathies can also be seen in diabetes. The most commonly involved nerves are ones that supply the extraocular muscles: especially CN III (oculomotor), VI (abducens), and IV (trochlear). Typical diabetic third-nerve palsy presents with unilateral pain, ptosis, and diplopia. Characteristically, there is sparing of pupillary function, but all patients with a third-nerve palsy should be carefully evaluated for a cerebral aneurysm.

Treatment-Induced Neuropathy of Diabetes

Treatment-induced neuropathy of diabetes is an acute, painful small-fiber neuropathy that is seen in patients with chronic hyperglycemia following a rapid improvement in glycemic control.[37] The severe neuropathic pain is often resistant to treatment and is frequently accompanied by autonomic symptoms that may include orthostatic hypotension, changes in sweating, gastroparesis, or erectile dysfunction. Patients with T1DM are at a higher risk of developing treatment-induced neuropathy of diabetes, and the severity of neuropathy is linked to the magnitude of change in the HbA_{1c}. The exact underlying cause of this disorder is unknown. There is evidence of a diffuse microvascular process with worsening of retinopathy and nephropathy along with the neuropathy. Patients with a history of diabetic anorexia, which is purposefully withholding insulin for weight loss, are at a higher risk of developing treatment-induced neuropathy of diabetes. Management is symptomatic, and one can expect improvement over time with ongoing stable glucose control. It is recommended to stabilize the current HbA_{1c} until symptoms improve and avoid labile glucose control by limiting changes in HbA_{1c} to 1% per month.

Diabetic neuropathic cachexia is a related disorder that also causes an acute painful diabetic neuropathy. It presents with widespread neuropathic pain that typically affects the trunk in addition to the limbs. It is accompanied by significant unintentional weight loss and is due to an acute diabetic polyradiculopathy that is superimposed on a severe peripheral neuropathy. Diabetic neuropathic cachexia is typically seen in middle-aged men with T2DM on oral hypoglycemic agents. Treatment is supportive, and most patients improve spontaneously within 1 to 2 years, although there may be residual deficits.

SUMMARY

Diabetic neuropathy is a common disorder with a diverse presentation. Improvement in glycemic control, lipids, blood pressure, and smoking cessation along with an earlier diagnosis and intervention have all helped to reduce the severity and slow the progression of diabetic neuropathy. There is evidence from natural history studies to suggest that diet and exercise interventions may reduce the progression of neuropathy or possibly even result in the regrowth of the epidermal nerve fibers.[24] Other clinical intervention studies have thus far not shown that a specific pharmacologic approach can reverse or prevent diabetic neuropathy. However, in the treatment of neuropathic pain, there has been greater success, and all patients with diabetic neuropathy should be counseled in foot care and fall prevention.

CLINICS CARE POINTS

- Approximately 50% of patients with diabetes will develop neuropathy.
- Patients with an otherwise idiopathic neuropathy should be screened with an oral glucose tolerance test and HgBA1c.
- Atypical features in a patient with suspected distal symmetric polyneuropathy include significant asymmetry, acute onset, rapid progression, or early motor involvement.
- Strict glucose control has been shown to prevent and improve neuropathy in type 1 diabetes, but there is less convincing evidence in type 2 diabetes.
- In addition to hyperglycemia, the components of the metabolic syndrome (dyslipidemia, hypertension, obesity) contribute to the risk of neuropathy in type 2 diabetes.
- Diabetic cardiovascular autonomic neuropathy is associated with an increased risk of mortality.
- The initial evaluation of orthostatic hypotension should include a comprehensive review of medications that may be contributing.
- Gastroparesis can cause difficult-to-control diabetes because of delayed intestinal absorption of glucose.
- Diabetic lumbosacral radiculoplexus neuropathy typically presents with acute onset of pain and weakness in the proximal leg of a diabetic patient.
- Treatment-induced neuropathy of diabetes typically presents with an acute painful small-fiber neuropathy in a diabetic patient with a preceding significant improvement in glycemic control.

DISCLOSURE

Dr. L. A. Zilliox have received funding from the Department of Veterans Affairs (Grant ID IK2RX001651).

REFERENCES

1. IDF. IDF diabetes Atlasvol. 7. Brussels (Belgium): International Diabetes Federation; 2015. p. 1–144. Available at: http://www.diabetesatlas.org.
2. Ziegler D. Cardiovascular autonomic neuropathy: clinical manifestations and measurement. Diabetes Rev 1999;7:342–57.
3. Schofield CJ, Libby G, Brennan GM, et al. Mortality and hospitalization in patients after amputation: a comparison between patients with and without diabetes. Diabetes Care 2006;29(10):2252–6.
4. Cohen JA, Jeffers BW, Faldut D, et al. Risks for sensorimotor peripheral neuropathy and autonomic neuropathy in non-insulin-dependent diabetes mellitus (NIDDM). Muscle Nerve 1998;21:72–80.
5. Smith AG, Singleton JR. The diagnostic yield of a standardized approach to idiopathic sensory-predominant neuropathy. Arch Intern Med 2004;164(9):1021–5.
6. Bongaerts BW, Rathmann W, Kowall B, et al. Postchallenge hyperglycemia is positively associated with diabetic polyneuropathy: the KORA F4 study. Diabetes Care 2012;35(9):1891–3.
7. Pop-Busui R, Boulton AJ, Feldman EL, et al. Diabetic neuropathy: a position statement by the American Diabetes Association. Diabetes Care 2017;40(1): 136–54.
8. Singleton JR, Smith AG, Russell JW, et al. Polyneuropathy with impaired glucose tolerance: implications for diagnosis and therapy. Curr Treat Options Neurol 2004; 7:33–42.
9. Tesfaye S, Chaturvedi N, Eaton SE, et al. Vascular risk factors and diabetic neuropathy. N Engl J Med 2005;352(4):341–50.
10. Costa LA, Canani LH, Lisbôa HR, et al. Aggregation of features of the metabolic syndrome is associated with increased prevalence of chronic complications in type 2 diabetes. Diabet Med 2004;21(3):252–5.
11. Callaghan BC, Xia R, Banerjee M, et al. Metabolic syndrome components are associated with symptomatic polyneuropathy independent of glycemic status. Diabetes Care 2016;39(5):801–7.
12. Schlesinger S, Herder C, Kannenberg JM, et al. General and abdominal obesity and incident distal sensorimotor polyneuropathy: insights into inflammatory biomarkers as potential mediators in the KORA F4/FF4 Cohort. Diabetes Care 2019;42(2):240–7.
13. Eid S, Sas KM, Abcouwer SF, et al. New insights into the mechanisms of diabetic complications: role of lipids and lipid metabolism. Diabetologia 2019;62(9): 1539–49.
14. Smith AG, Rose K, Singleton JR. Idiopathic neuropathy patients are at high risk for metabolic syndrome. J Neurol Sci 2008;273(1–2):25–8.
15. Malik RA. Pathology of human diabetic neuropathy. Handb Clin Neurol 2014;126: 249–59.
16. Kennedy JM, Zochodne DW. Impaired peripheral nerve regeneration in diabetes mellitus. J Peripher Nerv Syst 2005;10(2):144–57.
17. Ismail-Beigi F, Craven T, Banerji MA, et al. Effect of intensive treatment of hyperglycaemia on microvascular outcomes in type 2 diabetes: an analysis of the ACCORD randomised trial. Lancet 2010;376(9739):419–30.
18. Intensive blood-glucose control with sulphonylureas or insulin compared with conventional treatment and risk of complications in patients with type 2 diabetes (UKPDS 33). UK Prospective Diabetes Study (UKPDS) Group. Lancet 1998; 352(9131):837–53.

19. Group DR. The effect of intensive diabetes therapy on the development and progression of neuropathy. Ann Intern Med 1995;122:561–8.
20. Martin CL, Albers JW, Pop-Busui R. Neuropathy and related findings in the diabetes control and complications trial/epidemiology of diabetes interventions and complications study. Diabetes Care 2014;37(1):31–8.
21. Pop-Busui R, Lu J, Brooks MM, et al. Impact of glycemic control strategies on the progression of diabetic peripheral neuropathy in the Bypass Angioplasty Revascularization Investigation 2 Diabetes (BARI 2D) Cohort. Diabetes Care 2013; 36(10):3208–15.
22. Knowler WC, Barrett-Connor E, Fowler SE, et al. Reduction in the incidence of type 2 diabetes with lifestyle intervention or metformin. N Engl J Med 2002; 346(6):393–403.
23. Group DPPR. Long-term effects of lifestyle intervention or metformin on diabetes development and microvascular complications over 15-year follow-up: the Diabetes Prevention Program Outcomes Study. Lancet Diabetes Endocrinol 2015; 3(11):866–75.
24. Smith AG, Russell J, Feldman EL, et al. Lifestyle intervention for pre-diabetic neuropathy. Diabetes Care 2006;29(6):1294–9.
25. Singleton JR, Marcus RL, Jackson JE, et al. Exercise increases cutaneous nerve density in diabetic patients without neuropathy. Ann Clin Transl Neurol 2014; 1(10):844–9.
26. Singleton JR, Marcus RL, Lessard MK, et al. Supervised exercise improves cutaneous reinnervation capacity in metabolic syndrome patients. Ann Neurol 2015; 77(1):146–53.
27. American Diabetes A. 2. Classification and diagnosis of diabetes: standards of medical care in diabetes-2018. Diabetes Care 2018;41(Suppl 1):S13–27.
28. Kluding PM, Pasnoor M, Singh R, et al. The effect of exercise on neuropathic symptoms, nerve function, and cutaneous innervation in people with diabetic peripheral neuropathy. J Diabetes Complications 2012;26(5):424–9.
29. Bril V, England J, Franklin GM, et al. Evidence-based guideline: treatment of painful diabetic neuropathy: report of the American Academy of Neurology, the American Association of Neuromuscular and Electrodiagnostic Medicine, and the American Academy of Physical Medicine and Rehabilitation. Neurology 2011; 76(20):1758–65.
30. Ziegler D, Ametov A, Barinov A, et al. Oral treatment with alpha-lipoic acid improves symptomatic diabetic polyneuropathy: the SYDNEY 2 trial. Diabetes Care 2006;29(11):2365–70.
31. Ziegler D, Low PA, Litchy WJ, et al. Efficacy and safety of antioxidant treatment with alpha-lipoic acid over 4 years in diabetic polyneuropathy: the NATHAN 1 trial. Diabetes Care 2011;34(9):2054–60.
32. Lewis EJH, Perkins BA, Lovblom LE, et al. Effect of omega-3 supplementation on neuropathy in type 1 diabetes: a 12-month pilot trial. Neurology 2017;88(24): 2294–301.
33. Zilliox L, Peltier AC, Wren PA, et al. Assessing autonomic dysfunction in early diabetic neuropathy: the Survey of Autonomic Symptoms. Neurology 2011;76(12): 1099–105.
34. The Diabetes Control and Complications Trial Research Group. The effect of intensive diabetes therapy on measures of autonomic nervous system function in the Diabetes Control and Complications Trial (DCCT). Diabetologia 1998; 41(4):416–23.

35. Uddin SMI, Mirbolouk M, Dardari Z, et al. Erectile dysfunction as an independent predictor of future cardiovascular events: the multi-ethnic study of atherosclerosis. Circulation 2018;138(5):540–2.
36. Dyck PJ, Norell JE. Methylprednisolone may improve lumbosacral radiculoplexus neuropathy. Can J Neurol Sci 2001;28(3):224–7.
37. Gibbons CH, Freeman R. Treatment-induced neuropathy of diabetes: an acute, iatrogenic complication of diabetes. Brain 2015;138(Pt 1):43–52.

When Is It Not Diabetic Neuropathy? Atypical Peripheral Neuropathies, Neurologic Mimics, and Laboratory Work-up

Peter H. Jin, MD

KEYWORDS

- Neuropathy • Diabetes • Laboratory workup • Differential diagnosis

KEY POINTS

- Understanding the fundamental components of a typical chronic, sensory, length-dependent peripheral neuropathy is essential to proper diagnostic recognition of atypical peripheral neuropathies.
- Due to the nonspecific features of peripheral neuropathy, there are many other neurologic mimics.
- Laboratory work-up of etiologies of peripheral neuropathy should focus on high-yield tests and individual risk factors.

INTRODUCTION

The clinical presentation of peripheral neuropathy (also known as polyneuropathy) can be nonspecific. Many of the symptoms that patients report with peripheral neuropathy may be present in other neurologic diseases. Furthermore, not all peripheral neuropathies are equal in severity. Although most peripheral neuropathies are chronic and slowly progressive, there is a subset of peripheral neuropathies that are acute and aggressive and warrant urgent treatment. Different pathologies of peripheral neuropathies also can present nearly identically clinically, which can lead to challenges in identifying the etiology of a neuropathy. An understanding of red flags in patients with peripheral neuropathy symptoms along with how to begin a work-up for potential etiologies is fundamental to the management of peripheral neuropathy and its mimics.

Sources of funding: None.
Department of Neurology, University of Maryland School of Medicine, 110 South Paca Street, Third Floor, Baltimore, MD 21021, USA
E-mail address: pjin@som.umaryland.edu

WHAT ARE THE COMPONENTS OF TYPICAL DIABETIC NEUROPATHY?

Diabetic neuropathy (more formally known as diabetic sensory polyneuropathy) is the most common peripheral neuropathy disease that most geriatricians encounter. Breaking down this disease into its fundamental neurologic clinical components is helpful for several reasons. For one, it introduces the language used to describe peripheral neuropathies. Second, it establishes a baseline from which other neuropathies can be compared and can assist the clinician in determining if a patient's clinical presentation is atypical. Fundamentally, diabetic neuropathy is a chronic, slowly progressive, sensory-predominant, length-dependent peripheral neuropathy.

- Chronic and slowly progressive—patients do not seek medical attention until months to years after the onset of symptoms. The symptoms may worsen but only when evaluated over the course of months to years.
- Sensory predominant—the main symptoms and signs are related to sensory dysfunction. The symptoms may include paresthesia, numbness, and allodynia. The signs on examination may include decrease in pin or vibration sense and reduced deep tendon reflexes. Weakness is an uncommon complaint and rarely found on examination except in advanced cases.
- Length-dependent pattern—multiple terminal nerves are affected and nerves that are longer in their course are affected first. The pattern is symmetric, affecting both sides equally. The lower extremities should be affected before the upper extremities. Symptoms begin in the toes and feet.

This pattern of a chronic, sensory-predominant, length-dependent distribution is the most common pattern of peripheral neuropathies and generally portends a relatively benign syndrome. Other synonyms for this pattern include distal symmetric polyneuropathy, distal sensory polyneuropathy, and stocking-and-glove polyneuropathy.

TESTING FOR OTHER ETIOLOGIES OF CHRONIC, SENSORY-PREDOMINANT, LENGTH-DEPENDENT PERIPHERAL NEUROPATHY

Although diabetes is the most common etiology of chronic, sensory, length-dependent peripheral neuropathy, this pattern can be seen in neuropathy due to various other systemic diseases. Aside from diabetes, the most common etiologies include other metabolic disorders (uremia and hypothyroidism), medication toxicity (chemotherapy), nutritional deficiency, and alcohol toxicity. A thorough history and examination uncovers many of these etiologies (see Rajeev Motiwala's article, "A Clinical Approach to Disease of Peripheral Nerve," in this issue). Unfortunately, in many patients, the etiology of peripheral neuropathy is not clear based on history and examination alone. This is complicated further by how peripheral neuropathy can be the heralding finding of a systemic disease that precedes more classic symptoms and signs. More than 100 causes of neuropathy have been identified, and, as a result, diagnostic testing for neuropathy etiologies quickly can become very extensive and expensive.[1] Rather than testing for every possible cause of neuropathy, a measured approach is favored.

As a start, the American Academy of Neurology practice parameters recommend testing for fasting glucose, vitamin B_{12} deficiency, and monoclonal gammopathies as the highest yield tests for etiologies of peripheral neuropathy.[2] When screening for monoclonal gammopathy disorders, performing both serum protein electrophoresis and immunofixation increases sensitivity.[3] Beyond these tests, evidence-based guidance is limited. In my clinical practice, I routinely evaluate for common medical diseases where neuropathy can be the heralding sign.[4–7] If the initial laboratory evaluation is negative, I may send for more extensive laboratory testing based on clinical progression and results of electrodiagnostic testing (**Table 1**). Glucose intolerance diagnosed via a 2-hour oral glucose tolerance test has been identified as a frequently missed cause of what otherwise was thought to be idiopathic neuropathy. In spite of thorough testing, approximately 20% to 30% of patients with peripheral neuropathy do not have a determinable cause. Repeat laboratory and electrodiagnostic (EMG) testing may not yield additional information.[8,9] Some of these cases have been classified as chronic idiopathic axonal polyneuropathy, which typically has an age of onset of 50 years to 60 years, has a benign and slowly progressive course, and may be related to metabolic syndrome and oxidative stress.[10]

FEATURES OF ATYPICAL NEUROPATHY

Although a chronic, sensory-predominant, length-dependent pattern is typical for neuropathy, the opposite findings can be seen in atypical neuropathies. Atypical neuropathies can have a more acute onset, a non–length-dependent pattern of symptoms, and a more prominent motor component. The presence of any of these features should prompt consideration beyond typical neuropathies. In addition to the characteristics of the neuropathy, many atypical neuropathies also are accompanied by other systemic symptoms. Examples of atypical neuropathies include Guillain-Barre Syndrome, chronic inflammatory demyelinating polyradiculoneuropathy, vasculitis neuropathy and mononeuritis multiplex, hereditary neuropathies, and amyloid neuropathy. Diagnosis of these conditions usually requires a combination of second-line laboratory evaluation, electrodiagnostic testing, nerve biopsy, and/or genetic testing. Many of these disorders are discussed in Joseph M. Choi and Gianluca Di Maria's article, "Electrodiagnostic Testing for Disorders of Peripheral Nerves"; Natalia L. Gonzalez and Lisa D. Hobson-Webb's article, "The Role of Imaging for

Table 1
Laboratory testing for chronic, sensory, length-dependent peripheral neuropathies

Consider in all Patients	Consider in Select Patients Depending on Risk and Clinical Findings
Basic metabolic function panel with fasting glucose	2-h glucose tolerance test
Complete blood cell count	Methylmalonic acid
Liver function panel	Homocysteine level
Vitamin B_{12}	Vitamin E
Vitamin B_1	Vitamin B_6
Serum protein immunofixation electrophoresis	Copper
Thyroid function testing	Zinc
Antinuclear antigen	Human immunodeficiency virus
Sjögren syndrome antibodies A and B (anti-Ro, anti-La)	Lyme disease
	Hepatitis B and hepatitis C
	Cryoglobulin
	Rheumatoid factor
	Erythrocyte sedimentation rate
	C-reactive protein
	Antigliadin antibodies
	Anti–transglutaminase antibodies
	Antineutrophil cytoplasmic antibodies
	Serum light chains
	Urine immunofixation, electrophoresis, and light chains

Disorders of Peripheral Nerve"; and Stephen Cox and Kelly G. Gwathmey's article, "Chronic Immune-mediated Polyneuropathies," in this issue.

- Acute and rapidly progressive—severe degree of symptoms develops rapidly over a period of days to weeks. This pattern is the hallmark for Guillain-Barré syndrome, which can be considered an acute neuropathy. Neuropathy symptoms that occur acutely should prompt emergency neurologic evaluation (please see Justin Kwan and Suur Biliciler's article, "Guillain-Barre Syndrome and Other Acute Polyneuropathies," in this issue for further information).
- Motor prominent—motor symptoms are present beyond mild weakness in the toes. Muscle atrophy and fasciculations may be present. The patient may complain of falls or dropping objects. Some diseases may be motor predominant or pure motor, where sensory findings are limited or nonexistent. Motor prominent patterns are important to recognize because they can be seen in serious conditions, including amyotrophic lateral sclerosis, myasthenia gravis, myopathies, and rarely immune-mediated pure motor neuropathies. Among these diseases, clinical differentiation often is difficult, and EMG is necessary to establish a diagnosis. Expedited neurologic evaluation is warranted in these patients because several of these diagnoses are associated with early respiratory dysfunction.
- Non–length-dependent pattern—multiple nerves are affected, but both proximal and distal nerves are involved. There also may be asymmetry of findings. This pattern is seen in many different neuropathies. The most common diagnosis often is multiple compression mononeuropathies, where a patient may have multiple focal neuropathies at compression sites that give the appearance of a more diffuse peripheral neuropathy. For example, a patient with bilateral ulnar neuropathy at the elbow may have symptoms of bilateral hand tingling without symptoms in feet and may be mistaken as having a peripheral neuropathy. More rarely, peripheral neuropathies can be non–length dependent and affect nerves in an indiscriminate pattern. The classic example is mononeuritis multiplex secondary to vasculitis, where there is dysfunction in multiple unrelated nerves in a random distribution, which often leads to a patchy pattern of symptoms. This is in contrast to the length-dependent stocking-and-glove pattern.
- Associated systemic symptoms—various non-neurologic clinical features are found in atypical neuropathies. Many of these are related to the rheumatologic and inflammatory nature of these disorders. Symptoms and signs to inquire about include B symptoms (eg, fever, chills, and weight loss), skin changes, joint inflammation, and prominent autonomic symptoms (eg, orthostatic hypotension, early satiety, diarrhea, constipation, and erectile dysfunction).[11]

CLINICAL PATTERNS OF NON-NEUROPATHY NEUROLOGIC MIMICS

In addition to recognizing deviations from the fundamental components of common peripheral neuropathy, it also is helpful to understand specific features of other neurologic localizations. Many neurologic disorders have some form of disturbance of sensation, motor function, and balance. The presence of these symptoms is nonspecific to neuropathy because they can be caused by dysfunction in other parts of the nervous system. Determining which part of the nervous system is the generator of dysfunction (otherwise known as the localizing the lesion) is a fundamental skill for neurologic diagnosis and is required for diagnostic accuracy of neuropathy. This often is accomplished with determining if there are findings less typical for neuropathy and more typical for another localization. For example, the presence of hyperreflexia is an

Table 2
Neurologic localization mimics of peripheral neuropathy

Localization	Common Etiologies in Geriatrics	Potential Similar Findings that May Lead to Mistaken Diagnosis of Peripheral Neuropathy	Potential Distinguishing Features Compared with Peripheral Neuropathy
Brain and brainstem	Stroke, neoplasm, multiple sclerosis	• May have predominantly distal motor and sensory symptoms	• Alteration in mental status • Cranial nerve dysfunction • Cerebellar dysfunction • Usually unilateral and may have a hemibody pattern of involvement
Spinal cord (myelopathy)	Degenerative disk and joint disease of the cervical spine[13]	• Sensory and motor findings can be predominantly seen in lower extremities and be mistaken for a length-dependent pattern. • Frequently have bilateral symptoms	• Upper motor neuron findings (eg, hyperreflexia, and spasticity) • Sensory level loss (eg, diffuse sensory loss below the level of the C8 dermatome) • Bowel and bladder dysfunction • Saddle anesthesia
Spinal root (radiculopathy)	Degenerative disk and joint disease of cervical and lumbar spine[14]	• Certain dermatomal and myotomal patterns can appear like a distal pattern, for example, C8 radiculopathy presenting as hand weakness and fourth and fifth digit numbness.	• Sensory symptoms usually have a radiating quality from proximal region (neck, shoulder, or hip) to down the limb. • More often unilateral • Sensory loss involves a dermatomal distribution (eg, C8 dermatome). • Weakness involves a myotomal distribution (eg, C8 innervated muscles, which includes both the ulnar and median nerves).

(continued on next page)

Table 2
(continued)

Localization	Common Etiologies in Geriatrics	Potential Similar Findings that May Lead to Mistaken Diagnosis of Peripheral Neuropathy	Potential Distinguishing Features Compared with Peripheral Neuropathy
Anterior horn cell (motor neuron disease)	Amyotrophic lateral sclerosis[15]	• Weakness may be predominantly distal on initial presentation.	• Pure motor syndrome—sensory deficits on examination are limited or nonexistent. • In amyotrophic lateral sclerosis, there is presence of both upper and lower motor neuron findings. • Bulbar findings (eg, facial weakness, dysphagia, and dysarthria).
Dorsal root ganglion (sensory neuronopathy)	Sjögren disease, cisplatin chemotherapy, anti-Hu paraneoplastic syndrome, vitamin B_6 toxicity[16]	• Prominent sensory findings that may involve distal limb	• Sensory findings often are asymmetric and have a patchy and non–length-dependent pattern. • More pronounced deficit in proprioception (joint position sense, positive Romberg, sensory ataxia)
Neuromuscular junction	Myasthenia gravis, Lambert-Eaton myasthenic syndrome[17]	• Weakness may be predominantly distal.	• Pure motor syndrome—sensory deficits on examination are limited or nonexistent. • Oculomotor dysfunction and ptosis are common. • Weakness is fatigable and worse later on in the day.

(continued on next page)

Localization	Common Etiologies in Geriatrics	Potential Similar Findings that May Lead to Mistaken Diagnosis of Peripheral Neuropathy	Potential Distinguishing Features Compared with Peripheral Neuropathy
Table 2 (*continued*)			
Muscle (myopathy)	Dermatomyositis, inclusion body myositis, steroid myopathy[18,19]	• Certain myopathies can present with distal weakness (namely, inclusion body myositis with finger flexor weakness). • Muscle ache and cramping can be mistaken for sensory dysfunction.	• Pure motor syndrome—sensory deficits on examination are limited or nonexistent. • Most common pattern is proximal weakness (shoulder or hip).

upper motor neuron sign that should not be present in neuropathy. Its presence should lead the clinician to consider localizations of the brain or spinal cord more strongly than neuropathy. Another example is the presence of cranial nerve dysfunction, which should lead the clinician to consider potential localizations in the brainstem. Patterns of symptom distribution also can be helpful. For example, a patient with sensory disturbance in a hemibody distribution should lead the clinician to consider localizations in the brain or spinal cord more strongly than neuropathy. Some localizations have more nuanced differentiations from neuropathy and may require electrodiagnostic testing to distinguish. Examples include sensory neuronopathies, which may present exclusively with sensory findings but is distinguished by prominent proprioception deficits and asymmetric electrodiagnostic findings. Common neurologic mimics of peripheral neuropathy along with comparative features are briefly described in **Table 2**. An in-depth discussion of these diseases is beyond the scope of this article.

SHOULD ELECTRODIAGNOSTIC TESTING BE ORDERED FOR NEUROPATHY?

In cases of suspected atypical neuropathy, EMG always is warranted. In patients with clear, length-dependent, chronically progressive, predominantly sensory neuropathy, EMG may be warranted. A common rationale for deferring EMG is that the test simply confirms the clinical diagnosis, and management of the disease does not change. Various studies, however, have demonstrated that EMG testing of patients with classic peripheral neuropathy can change management, change diagnosis, or provide additional diagnoses.[12] This is not surprising given the many diagnostic mimics and nuances of neuropathy. Patients also may have multiple neurologic diagnoses that contribute to their symptoms, which EMG can help elucidate.

CLINICAL CARE POINTS—FEATURES OF ATYPICAL NEUROPATHIES THAT SHOULD PROMPT NEUROLOGY CONSULTATION

- Acute or subacute progression
- Weakness beyond mild distal weakness

- Patchy distribution of sensory findings
- Prominent autonomic symptoms
- B symptoms
- Skin changes
- Joint inflammation

CLINICAL CARE POINTS—FEATURES OF NEUROLOGIC MIMICS OF NEUROPATHY THAT SHOULD PROMPT NEUROLOGY CONSULTATION

- Alterations in consciousness or cognition
- Cranial nerve dysfunction
- Cerebellar dysfunction
- Prominent proprioception deficits
- Upper motor neuron findings
- Motor-predominant syndromes

SUMMARY

A large majority of peripheral neuropathies that geriatricians encounter are typical peripheral neuropathies. Due to their nonspecific symptoms, however, there are many diseases that present similarly. An understanding of the fundamental components of neuropathy along with distinguishing features of clinical mimics can lead providers to a more confident diagnosis of a typical peripheral neuropathy or to consider other diagnostic possibilities. In patients with neuropathy without obvious cause, a measured and case-by-case work-up can uncover other etiologies of neuropathy.

ACKNOWLEDGMENTS

None.

DISCLOSURE

The author has nothing to disclose.

REFERENCES

1. Mauermann ML, Burns TM. The evaluation of chronic axonal polyneuropathies. Semin Neurol 2008;28(2):133–51.
2. England JD, Gronseth GS, Franklin G, et al. Practice parameter: evaluation of distal symmetric polyneuropathy: role of laboratory and genetic testing (an evidence-based review): report of the American academy of neurology, American association of neuromuscular and electrodiagnostic medicine, and American academy of physical medicine and rehabilitation. Neurology 2009;72(2):185–92.
3. Katzmann JA. Screening panels for monoclonal gammopathies: time to change. Clin Biochem Rev 2009;30(3):105–11. Available at: http://www.ncbi.nlm.nih.gov/pubmed/19841692. Accessed June 17, 2020.
4. Lang M, Treister R, Oaklander AL. Diagnostic value of blood tests for occult causes of initially idiopathic small-fiber polyneuropathy. J Neurol 2016;263(12):2515–27.
5. Laurikka P, Nurminen S, Kivelä L, et al. Extraintestinal manifestations of celiac disease: early detection for better long-term outcomes. Nutrients 2018;10(8). https://doi.org/10.3390/nu10081015.

6. Siekert RG, Clark EC. Neurologic signs and symptoms as early manifestations of systemic lupus erythematosus. Neurology 1955;5(2):84–8.
7. Gemignani F, Marbini A, Pavesi G, et al. Peripheral neuropathy associated with primary Sjögren's syndrome. J Neurol Neurosurg Psychiatry 1994;57(8):983–6.
8. Lau KHV. Laboratory evaluation of peripheral neuropathy. Semin Neurol 2019; 39(5):531–41.
9. Jann S, Beretta S, Bramerio M, et al. Prospective follow-up study of chronic poly-neuropathy of undetermined cause. Muscle Nerve 2001;24(9):1197–201.
10. Singer MA, Vernino SA, Wolfe GI. Idiopathic neuropathy: new paradigms, new promise. J Peripher Nerv Syst 2012;17(SUPPL. 2):43–9.
11. Karam C, Tramontozzi LA. Rapid screening for inflammatory neuropathies by standardized clinical criteria. Neurol Clin Pract 2016;6(5):384–8.
12. Bodofsky EB, Carter GT, England JD. Is electrodiagnosic testing for polyneurop-athy overutilized? Muscle Nerve 2017;55(3):301–4.
13. Toledano M, Bartleson JD. Cervical spondylotic myelopathy. Neurol Clin 2013; 31(1):287–305.
14. Iyer S, Kim HJ. Cervical radiculopathy. Curr Rev Musculoskelet Med 2016;9(3): 272–80.
15. van Es MA, Hardiman O, Chio A, et al. Amyotrophic lateral sclerosis. Lancet 2017;390(10107):2084–98.
16. Gwathmey KG. Sensory neuronopathies. Muscle Nerve 2016;53(1):8–19.
17. Gilhus NE. Myasthenia gravis. N Engl J Med 2016;375(26):2570–81.
18. Greenberg SA. Inclusion body myositis: clinical features and pathogenesis. Nat Rev Rheumatol 2019;15(5):257–72.
19. Clark KEN, Isenberg DA. A review of inflammatory idiopathic myopathy focusing on polymyositis. Eur J Neurol 2018;25(1):13–23.

Small Fiber Neuropathy in the Elderly

Lan Zhou, MD, PhD

KEYWORDS

- Small fiber neuropathy • Elderly • Clinical features • Management

KEY POINTS

- Small fiber neuropathy (SFN) is common and prevalent in the elderly.
- SFN typically manifests as pain, burning, tingling, and numbness in the feet and hands.
- Skin biopsy with intraepidermal nerve fiber density evaluation is the gold standard diagnostic test.
- SFN can be associated with many medical conditions, with diabetes mellitus the most common.
- Treatment should be individualized to control underlying causes, alleviate pain, and optimize function.

Small fiber neuropathy (SFN) is a type of peripheral neuropathy that solely or predominantly affects small myelinated Aδ fibers and unmyelinated C fibers. The disease is common and can be associated with many medical conditions, including diabetes mellitus, connective tissue diseases, sarcoidosis, vitamin B_{12} deficiency, monoclonal gammopathy, thyroid dysfunction, human immunodeficiency virus (HIV) and hepatitis C virus (HCV) infections, sodium channelopathy, metabolic syndrome, and paraneoplastic syndrome, among others.[1–10] SFN is more prevalent in the elderly than in younger adults. According to a Dutch study, the minimum prevalence of SFN is 52.95 per 100,000 population, with the rates higher in elderly patients compared with younger patients.[11] Another cohort study from Netherlands showed that among 598 patients who were diagnosed with SFN, 117 (19.6%) were 65 years or older.[12] Age is an independent risk factor for SFN.[13] Although aging may play a role in small fiber degeneration, the increase in the prevalence of diabetes mellitus, metabolic syndrome, and monoclonal gammopathy also likely contributes to the higher prevalence of SFN in the elderly. SFN often has a negative impact on quality of life, both physically and mentally, due to annoying neuropathic pain.[14] Pain control can be challenging particularly in elderly patients due to safety and tolerability of

The author has nothing to disclose.
Department of Neurology, Boston Medical Center Cutaneous Nerve Laboratory, Boston University School of Medicine, 72 East Concord Street, Boston, MA 02118, USA
E-mail address: lanzhou@bu.edu

medications. Early diagnosis and individualized treatment are important for controlling SFN and optimizing daily function in this patient population. This article reviews clinical features, diagnostic evaluation, etiology evaluation, management, and prognosis of SFN, with a focus on the elderly.

CLINICAL FEATURES

SFN can affect somatic sensory fibers and autonomic C fibers. Most patients have predominant somatic involvement. Small somatic sensory fibers innervate skin to control the perception of pinprick and thermal stimuli. Loss of these fibers can cause numbness to pinprick and temperature. Ectopic firing of these fibers or hyperexcitability of dorsal root ganglia that give rise to these fibers can cause pain, burning, and tingling sensation.[15] Patients also may report squeeze sensation, coldness, or itchy skin in the affected areas.[16,17] These sensory symptoms usually are worse at night. SFN often is painful, especially when associated with amyloidosis, diabetes mellitus, HIV infection, sarcoidosis, sodium channelopathy, alcohol toxicity, and neurotoxic drug exposure, but it also can be nonpainful.[18,19] Examination may show allodynia (nonpainful stimuli perceived as painful), hyperalgesias (painful stimuli perceived as more painful than expected), and reduced pinprick and thermal sensation in the affected areas. Motor strength, proprioception, and deep tendon reflexes usually are preserved, because these are the functions of large fibers. Reduced vibratory sensation at toes and decreased deep tendon reflexes at ankles, however, may be detected in elderly patients with SFN, because these findings are not uncommon in older people without neuropathy.

SFN mostly is length-dependent (LD), with the most distal sites affected the first and the most. The common initial symptoms are burning feet and numb toes. The sensory symptoms then progress gradually to involve distal legs, fingers, and hands and eventually display a stocking-glove pattern.[1] Non–LD (NLD)-SFN is relatively rare, accounting for 20% to 25% of cases of pure SFN.[3,16] Sensory symptoms and signs in NLD-SFN usually are patchy, asymmetric, migrating, or diffuse, often involving trunk and face in addition to limbs.[3] Compared with LD-SFN, NLD-SFN is seen more commonly in woman with a younger age at onset and a higher association with immune-mediated conditions.[3,20,21] If elderly patients develop NLD-SFN, small sensory ganglionopathy should be considered, which can be associated with Sjögren's syndrome, sarcoidosis, and paraneoplastic syndrome.[3,22,23]

Autonomic C fibers innervate involuntary muscles, including cardiac muscle and smooth muscle. Smooth muscle is present in blood vessel walls, gastrointestinal tract, genitourinary tract, lacrimal gland, salivary gland, and sweat gland. Autonomic C fibers control cardiac muscle contractility, blood vessel constriction and dilatation, gastrointestinal and genitourinary motilities, and gland functions. Dysfunction of autonomic C fibers can cause palpitations, orthostatic dizziness, skin discoloration, bowel constipation and diarrhea, urinary retention, sexual dysfunction, dry eyes, dry mouth, and sweating abnormalities. When the disease is LD, patients may experience dry skin and reduced sweating in the feet (distal anhidrosis), due to impaired sudomotor autonomic function, but increased sweating in the trunk or face (compensatory proximal hyperhidrosis) to maintain thermoregulation. Examination may detect coldness and skin discoloration (white, red, or purple) in the feet and distal legs due to dysregulation of vasomotor autonomic functions.[1,15,19] When the disease is NLD, patients may develop dry eyes, dry mouth, palpitations, orthostatic dizziness, bowel constipation, and urinary retention.[19] Autonomic involvement frequently is seen in SFN associated with amyloidosis, diabetes mellitus, sarcoidosis, and Sjögren's syndrome. It can impair quality of life significantly. Dizziness may affect gait and lead to falls in elderly patients.

DIAGNOSTIC EVALUATION

Diagnosis of distal SFN is based on symptoms, signs, and diagnostic test findings. Routine nerve conduction study (NCS)/electromyography (EMG) typically is normal in patients with pure SFN, because the test evaluates only large fiber functions. NCS/EMG still should be done first, however, to rule out a large fiber polyneuropathy and bilateral S1 radiculopathies, which also can cause paresthesia in the feet, especially in elderly patients with low back pain. It is not uncommon for patients to have mixed large fiber and small fiber polyneuropathy. If a large fiber polyneuropathy is detected by NCS/EMG, skin biopsy is not needed, because a diagnosis of peripheral neuropathy is established. NCS may not be helpful for the diagnosis of distal sensory polyneuropathy in patients over age 75, because absent sural sensory responses can be attributed to aging changes.[24] Skin biopsy is useful to confirm distal sensory polyneuropathy in this age group.

Skin biopsy is the gold standard for diagnosing SFN with a high diagnostic efficiency.[25–28] It is useful for diagnosing not only LD-SFN but also NLD-SFN[3,16,20,21,29,30] and focal SFN, such as diabetic truncal neuropathy, meralgia paresthetica, and complex regional pain syndrome.[31–34] The 3-mm punch skin biopsy is an office procedure, easy to perform and minimally invasive. Biopsy is taken routinely from the distal leg, which is 7 cm to 10 cm above the lateral malleolus. Additional biopsies may be taken from distal thigh (7–10 cm above the knee) and proximal thigh (7–10 cm below the greater trochanter) for evaluation of the severity and pattern of SFN.[3,16,21,30] Biopsies may be taken from other sites if focal or unilateral small fiber impairment is suspected of affecting these sites.[31–34] Biopsy specimens should be sent to a diagnostic cutaneous nerve laboratory for processing and reading. A diagnosis of SFN is made if intraepidermal nerve fiber density (IENFD) is reduced. The age-adjusted and sex-adjusted worldwide normative values of IENFD at the distal leg have been established for clinical use.[35] The diagnostic sensitivity of using the normative values for elderly patients, however, has not been well studied. A recent small-scale study showed that IENFD at the distal leg appeared influenced by ethnicity.[36] Future studies are needed to fully address the ethnic differences in IENFD, and to adjust normative values to improve diagnostic sensitivity.

Quantitative sensory testing has been validated for evaluating symptoms of sensory neuropathy. The test has significant limitations, however.[37] It cannot differentiate whether impaired response to sensory stimuli is due to a peripheral nerve disease or to a central nervous system disorder, because a proper response requires an intact sensory pathway. The test requires cooperation of patients, and a slow response can result from cognitive deficit, poor concentration, or malingering. It is not recommended as a stand-alone test for SFN.[38]

Autonomic testing is helpful to evaluate neuropathy patients with autonomic symptoms. The quantitative sudomotor axon reflex test (QSART) evaluates postganglionic sympathetic unmyelinated sudomotor nerve function.[39] It may be ordered if patients have sweating abnormalities. QSART and skin biopsy combined can increase the diagnostic sensitivity of SFN.[22,40] QSART, however, is not widely available. The test is very sensitive to antihistamines and antidepressants because these medications may affect sweating. These medications should be discontinued 48 hours prior to the study. Cardiovascular autonomic testing is useful to evaluate patients with cardiovascular autonomic symptoms, such as orthostatic intolerance, palpitations, and tachycardia.

ETIOLOGY EVALUATION

SFN can be associated with many medical conditions, which can be identified in approximately half of cases.[2,3,25] Diabetes mellitus appears the most common cause of SFN in United States.[3,41]

Immune-mediated conditions are seen more commonly in NLD-SFN than in LD-SFN.[3] The other associated conditions include vitamin B_{12} deficiency, thyroid dysfunction, monoclonal gammopathy, metabolic syndrome, celiac disease, HIV and HCV infections, alcohol abuse, neurotoxic drug exposure, sodium channelopathy, amyloidosis, Fabry disease, and paraneoplastic syndrome.[1–10]

Thorough history taking is important and can help identify or raise suspicion for certain associated conditions, such as metabolic syndrome, alcohol abuse, neurotoxic drug exposure, HIV and HCV infections, and genetic causes. Alcohol toxicity and thallium poisoning can cause painful SFN.[42–44] Some neurotoxic drugs are more likely to cause painful SFN than others. These drugs include antibiotics (metronidazole, nitrofurantoin, fluoroquinolone, and linezolid),[45–50] chemotherapeutic agents (bortezomib, thalidomide, and vincristine),[51,52] and tumor necrosis factor inhibitors.[53] Rapid improvement of glycemic control in diabetic patients also can induce acute painful neuropathy.[54,55] It usually occurs when the hemoglobin (Hb) A_{1C} level is reduced by 2 or more percentage points over a 3-month period of time. The pain is severe and refractory to the treatment, but it improves spontaneously after 12 months to 24 months.[54,55] A diagnosis can be made or suspected by history-taking.

A battery of blood tests, including complete blood cell count, comprehensive metabolic panel, HbA_{1C}, lipid panel, thyroid-stimulating hormone, free thyroxine, erythrocyte sedimentation rate, antinuclear antibody, extractable nuclear antigens, immunofixation, and vitamin B_{12} and folate levels should be ordered to search for common etiologies of SFN; a 2-hour oral glucose tolerance test is more sensitive than HbA_{1C} and fasting glucose level for detecting diabetes and prediabetes in patients with SFN.[56] Additional tests may be ordered based on clinical history. HIV or HCV serology should be ordered if risk factors are present. Lip biopsy should be considered if clinical suspicion for Sjögren's syndrome or seronegative sicca syndrome is high. If amyloidosis is suspected, bone marrow or fat biopsy can be helpful. Skin biopsy also may show amyloid deposition.[57] Chest CT should be ordered if sarcoidosis is suspected.[58] If a history of gastrointestinal symptoms or gluten intolerance is present, gliadin antibody, tissue transglutaminase antibodies, and small bowel biopsy may be pursued to evaluate for celiac disease. Genetic testing should be considered if the disease onset is young and/or a positive family history is present. In a cohort of 1139 patients with pure SFN who were screened for sodium channelopathies, potential pathogenic variants of voltage-gated sodium channel genes, including SCN9A, SCN10A, and SCN11A, were detected in 132 (11.6%).[10] Genetic screening of Fabry disease in SFN patients is not cost-effective and should be done only if other clinical features are present.[4] Familial amyloidosis associated with transthyretin (TTR) gene mutations usually affects both large and small nerve fibers. It should be suspected if patients also have renal, cardiac, and hepatic abnormalities and bilateral carpal tunnel syndrome.[59]

MANAGEMENT

Management of SFN in the elderly consists of identifying and treating underlying causes, alleviating neuropathic pain, preventing injury, and optimizing daily function.

Etiology-specific treatment is the key to preventing or slowing down SFN progression. Diabetes mellitus and metabolic syndrome are more prevalent in the elderly than in younger patients. One study showed that metabolic syndrome was common in adults at or above 60 years of age in the United States, with the prevalence greater than 40%.[60] Metabolic syndrome consists of hypertension, glucose dysmetabolism, dyslipidemia, and central obesity. It is a significant risk factor not only for cardiovascular and cerebral vascular diseases but also for peripheral neuropathy, including pure SFN.[13] The link between metabolic syndrome and SFN is beyond glucose dysmetabolism, because the individual components of metabolic syndrome are independent risk factors.[13,61,62] Tight glycemic control and lifestyle modification with diet control, weight control, and regular exercise are important in patients with these conditions, which can help improve neuropathy symptoms and IENFD.[63,64] Rapid improvement of glycemic control, however, should be avoided in diabetic patients to prevent acute painful neuropathy. It has been reported that treatment of sarcoidosis, autoimmune diseases, vitamin B_{12} deficiency, and celiac disease improved symptoms of the SFN that resulted from these conditions.[19,22,65,66] In patients with SFN induced by alcohol abuse or neurotoxic drug exposure, cessation or avoidance of the toxic substance is beneficial for SFN symptoms.

Pain management is crucial in the treatment of SFN, because neuropathic pain is common in SFN and it often has a negative impact on quality of life, reducing physical activity and causing sleep deprivation and depression. Pain control can be particularly challenging in elderly patients, however, due to safety and tolerability of medications. Drug metabolism is slower in the elderly. Elderly patients also tend to have multiple comorbidities, such as hypertension and renal, hepatic, and cardiac dysfunctions.[12] As a result, the risk of adverse drug reactions is higher in the elderly. Elderly patients are more susceptible to drowsiness, dizziness, and other side effects from pain medications. Many of them take a list of other medications, which increases the risk of drug-drug interactions. These factors often limit the use of adequate doses of pain medications.[12,67–77] The types and doses of pain medications should be chosen carefully for elderly patients. Treatment should be individualized based on comorbidities, drug tolerability, and potential drug-drug interactions. For details on the treatment of neuropathic pain in the elderly, see the Elizabeth J. Pedowitz and colleagues' article, "Management of Neuropathic Pain in the Geriatric Population," in this issue.

Elderly patients with neuropathy symptoms are at a significant risk for physical injuries. Pain, numbness, dizziness, and drowsiness may cause gait imbalance and falls. Foot ulcers may develop, especially in patients with diabetes mellitus. Heat injury may occur in the feet and fingers due to numbness. Patients should be referred to physical therapy for gait training if gait abnormality is reported or detected. Wearing padded socks and supportive shoes can help foot protection and promote ulcer healing. Patients should be instructed to use emollient creams to moisturize dry skin and inspect the bottom of their feet with a mirror regularly for prevention and early detection of ulcer. Patients should test bath water with a body part without numbness before putting their feet in. They should be careful with cooking and should not sleep with feet close to a fireplace.[67] They should be encouraged to do exercise safely.

PROGNOSIS

Most patients with SFN experience a slowly progressive course. Two large cohort longitudinal studies showed that only a small percentage of these patients developed large fiber involvement over time, 11.9% in 1 study[41] and 13% in the other.[25] Most SFN patients, however, require chronic pain management. It is important to discuss with patients that the typical course of SFN is relatively benign because many of these patients often worry about developing weakness and loss of ambulation from the neuropathy. It also is important to explain to patients that the pain medications are used for controlling pain, burning, or tingling sensation but not numbness, because the numbness is caused by the loss of small fibers and the improvement relies on small fiber regeneration. There is no medication available at this point to promote nerve fiber regeneration. Numbness associated with mild SFN may improve, however, once the etiologies are controlled.[19,22,63–66]

SUMMARY

SFN is common and more prevalent in the elderly than in younger adults. It can have a negative impact on quality of life due to neuropathic pain, autonomic symptoms, and medication side effects. Skin biopsy with IENFD evaluation is the gold standard diagnostic test. Autonomic function testing is useful when autonomic symptoms are present. Screening for associated conditions should be done in every patient. Etiology-specific treatment, pain control, and injury prevention are the key elements of SFN management in the elderly. Pain management can be particularly challenging in elderly patients, and it should be individualized based on comorbidities, drug tolerability, and drug-drug interactions.

CLINICS CARE POINTS

- The hallmark features of SFN are numbness and tingling, sharp and burning pain, loss of pinprick and temperature sensation, and autonomic dysfunction. There is preservation of strength and joint position sense.
- Diabetes is the most common cause of SFN in the United States. Elderly age itself is a risk factor for SFN.
- Electrodiagnostic testing with NCS and EMG is normal in patients with SFN.
- The gold standard for diagnosis of SFN is skin biopsy with evaluation of IENFD.
- Treatment of SFN, similar to other neuropathies, is based on a combination of treating the underlying cause, neuropathic pain management, and lifestyle adjustments.
- Most patients with SFN have a benign course and do not develop subsequent difficulty with ambulation.

REFERENCES

1. Tavee J, Zhou L. Small fiber neuropathy: a burning problem. Cleve Clin J Med 2009;76(5):297–305.
2. de Greef BTA, Hoeijmakers JGJ, Gorissen-Brouwers CML, et al. Associated conditions in small fiber neuropathy - a large cohort study and review of the literature. Eur J Neurol 2018;25(2):348–55.
3. Khan S, Zhou L. Characterization of non-length-dependent small-fiber sensory neuropathy. Muscle Nerve 2012;45(1):86–91.
4. Cazzato D, Lauria G. Small fibre neuropathy. Curr Opin Neurol 2017;30(5):490–9.
5. Chan AC, Wilder-Smith EP. Small fiber neuropathy: getting bigger! Muscle Nerve 2016;53(5):671–82.
6. Zhou L. Small fiber neuropathy. Semin Neurol 2019;39(5):570–7.
7. Faber CG, Lauria G, Merkies IS, et al. Gain-of-function Nav1.8 mutations in painful neuropathy. Proc Natl Acad Sci U S A 2012;109(47):19444–9.

8. Hoeijmakers JG, Faber CG, Merkies IS, et al. Painful peripheral neuropathy and sodium channel mutations. Neurosci Lett 2015;596:51–9.
9. Huang J, Han C, Estacion M, et al. Gain-of-function mutations in sodium channel Na(v)1.9 in painful neuropathy. Brain 2014;137(Pt 6):1627–42.
10. Eijkenboom I, Sopacua M, Hoeijmakers JGJ, et al. Yield of peripheral sodium channels gene screening in pure small fibre neuropathy. J Neurol Neurosurg Psychiatry 2019;90(3):342–52.
11. Peters MJ, Bakkers M, Merkies IS, et al. Incidence and prevalence of small-fiber neuropathy: a survey in The Netherlands. Neurology 2013;81(15):1356–60.
12. Brouwer BA, de Greef BT, Hoeijmakers JG, et al. Neuropathic pain due to small fiber neuropathy in aging: current management and future prospects. Drugs Aging 2015;32(8):611–21.
13. Zhou L, Li J, Ontaneda D, et al. Metabolic syndrome in small fiber sensory neuropathy. J Clin Neuromuscul Dis 2011;12(4):235–43.
14. Bakkers M, Faber CG, Hoeijmakers JG, et al. Small fibers, large impact: quality of life in small-fiber neuropathy. Muscle Nerve 2014;49(3):329–36.
15. Lacomis D. Small-fiber neuropathy. Muscle Nerve 2002;26(2):173–88.
16. Gemignani F, Giovanelli M, Vitetta F, et al. Non-length dependent small fiber neuropathy. a prospective case series. J Peripher Nerv Syst 2010;15(1):57–62.
17. Misery L, Brenaut E, Le Garrec R, et al. Neuropathic pruritus. Nat Rev Neurol 2014;10(7):408–16.
18. Lauria G, Hsieh ST, Johansson O, et al. European Federation of Neurological Societies/Peripheral Nerve Society Guideline on the use of skin biopsy in the diagnosis of small fiber neuropathy. Report of a joint task force of the European Federation of Neurological Societies and the Peripheral Nerve Society. Eur J Neurol 2010;17(7):903–12, e944-909.
19. Gibbons CH. Small fiber neuropathies. Continuum (Minneap Minn) 2014;20(5 Peripheral Nervous System Disorders):1398–412.
20. Chai J, Herrmann DN, Stanton M, et al. Painful small-fiber neuropathy in Sjogren syndrome. Neurology 2005;65(6):925–7.
21. Gorson KC, Herrmann DN, Thiagarajan R, et al. Non-length dependent small fibre neuropathy/ganglionopathy. J Neurol Neurosurg Psychiatry 2008;79(2):163–9.
22. Tavee JO, Karwa K, Ahmed Z, et al. Sarcoidosis-associated small fiber neuropathy in a large cohort: clinical aspects and response to IVIG and anti-TNF alpha treatment. Respir Med 2017;126:135–8.
23. Descamps E, Henry J, Labeyrie C, et al. Small fiber neuropathy in Sjogren syndrome: comparison with other small fiber neuropathies. Muscle Nerve 2020; 61(4):515–20.
24. Tavee JO, Polston D, Zhou L, et al. Sural sensory nerve action potential, epidermal nerve fiber density, and quantitative sudomotor axon reflex in the healthy elderly. Muscle Nerve 2014;49(4):564–9.
25. Devigili G, Tugnoli V, Penza P, et al. The diagnostic criteria for small fibre neuropathy: from symptoms to neuropathology. Brain 2008;131(Pt 7):1912–25.
26. Lauria G, Holland N, Hauer P, et al. Epidermal innervation: changes with aging, topographic location, and in sensory neuropathy. J Neurol Sci 1999;164(2): 172–8.
27. McArthur JC, Stocks EA, Hauer P, et al. Epidermal nerve fiber density: normative reference range and diagnostic efficiency. Arch Neurol 1998;55(12):1513–20.
28. Vlckova-Moravcova E, Bednarik J, Dusek L, et al. Diagnostic validity of epidermal nerve fiber densities in painful sensory neuropathies. Muscle Nerve 2008;37(1): 50–60.

29. Lauria G, Sghirlanzoni A, Lombardi R, et al. Epidermal nerve fiber density in sensory ganglionopathies: clinical and neurophysiologic correlations. Muscle Nerve 2001;24(8):1034–9.

30. Provitera V, Gibbons CH, Wendelschafer-Crabb G, et al. The role of skin biopsy in differentiating small-fiber neuropathy from ganglionopathy. Eur J Neurol 2018; 25(6):848–53.

31. Chemali KR, Zhou L. Small fiber degeneration in post-stroke complex regional pain syndrome I. Neurology 2007;69(3):316–7.

32. Wongmek A, Shin S, Zhou L. Skin biopsy in assessing meralgia paresthetica. Muscle Nerve 2016;53(4):641–3.

33. Lauria G, McArthur JC, Hauer PE, et al. Neuropathological alterations in diabetic truncal neuropathy: evaluation by skin biopsy. J Neurol Neurosurg Psychiatry 1998;65(5):762–6.

34. Oaklander AL, Rissmiller JG, Gelman LB, et al. Evidence of focal small-fiber axonal degeneration in complex regional pain syndrome-I (reflex sympathetic dystrophy). Pain 2006;120(3):235–43.

35. Lauria G, Bakkers M, Schmitz C, et al. Intraepidermal nerve fiber density at the distal leg: a worldwide normative reference study. J Peripher Nerv Syst 2010; 15(3):202–7.

36. Jin P, Cheng L, Chen M, et al. Low sensitivity of skin biopsy in diagnosing small fiber neuropathy in Chinese Americans. J Clin Neuromuscul Dis 2018;20(1):1–6.

37. Backonja MM, Attal N, Baron R, et al. Value of quantitative sensory testing in neurological and pain disorders: NeuPSIG consensus. Pain 2013;154(9): 1807–19.

38. Shy ME, Frohman EM, So YT, et al. Quantitative sensory testing: report of the therapeutics and technology assessment subcommittee of the American Academy of Neurology. Neurology 2003;60(6):898–904.

39. Low VA, Sandroni P, Fealey RD, et al. Detection of small-fiber neuropathy by sudomotor testing. Muscle Nerve 2006;34(1):57–61.

40. Thaisetthawatkul P, Fernandes Filho JA, Herrmann DN. Contribution of QSART to the diagnosis of small fiber neuropathy. Muscle Nerve 2013;48(6):883–8.

41. MacDonald S, Sharma TL, Li J, et al. Longitudinal follow-up of biopsy-proven small fiber neuropathy. Muscle Nerve 2019;60(4):376–81.

42. Koike H, Mori K, Misu K, et al. Painful alcoholic polyneuropathy with predominant small-fiber loss and normal thiamine status. Neurology 2001;56(12):1727–32.

43. Kuo HC, Huang CC, Tsai YT, et al. Acute painful neuropathy in thallium poisoning. Neurology 2005;65(2):302–4.

44. Mellion ML, Silbermann E, Gilchrist JM, et al. Small-fiber degeneration in alcohol-related peripheral neuropathy. Alcohol Clin Exp Res 2014;38(7):1965–72.

45. Chao CC, Sun HY, Chang YC, et al. Painful neuropathy with skin denervation after prolonged use of linezolid. J Neurol Neurosurg Psychiatry 2008;79(1):97–9.

46. Heckmann JG, Dutsch M, Schwab S. Linezolid-associated small-fiber neuropathy. J Peripher Nerv Syst 2008;13(2):157–8.

47. Hobson-Webb LD, Roach ES, Donofrio PD. Metronidazole: newly recognized cause of autonomic neuropathy. J Child Neurol 2006;21(5):429–31.

48. Tan IL, Polydefkis MJ, Ebenezer GJ, et al. Peripheral nerve toxic effects of nitrofurantoin. Arch Neurol 2012;69(2):265–8.

49. Zivkovic SA, Lacomis D, Giuliani MJ. Sensory neuropathy associated with metronidazole: report of four cases and review of the literature. J Clin Neuromuscul Dis 2001;3(1):8–12.

50. Etminan M, Brophy JM, Samii A. Oral fluoroquinolone use and risk of peripheral neuropathy: a pharmacoepidemiologic study. Neurology 2014;83(14):1261–3.
51. Giannoccaro MP, Donadio V, Gomis Perez C, et al. Somatic and autonomic small fiber neuropathy induced by bortezomib therapy: an immunofluorescence study. Neurol Sci 2011;32(2):361–3.
52. Timmins HC, Li T, Kiernan MC, et al. Quantification of small fiber neuropathy in chemotherapy-treated patients. J Pain 2020;21(1–2):44–58.
53. Birnbaum J, Bingham CO 3rd. Non-length-dependent and length-dependent small-fiber neuropathies associated with tumor necrosis factor (TNF)-inhibitor therapy in patients with rheumatoid arthritis: expanding the spectrum of neurological disease associated with TNF-inhibitors. Semin Arthritis Rheum 2014;43(5):638–47.
54. Gibbons CH, Freeman R. Treatment-induced diabetic neuropathy: a reversible painful autonomic neuropathy. Ann Neurol 2010;67(4):534–41.
55. Gibbons CH, Freeman R. Treatment-induced neuropathy of diabetes: an acute, iatrogenic complication of diabetes. Brain 2015;138(Pt 1):43–52.
56. Sumner CJ, Sheth S, Griffin JW, et al. The spectrum of neuropathy in diabetes and impaired glucose tolerance. Neurology 2003;60(1):108–11.
57. Ebenezer GJ, Liu Y, Judge DP, et al. Cutaneous nerve biomarkers in transthyretin familial amyloid polyneuropathy. Ann Neurol 2017;82(1):44–56.
58. Tavee JO. Office approach to small fiber neuropathy. Cleve Clin J Med 2018;85(10):801–12.
59. Adams D, Suhr OB, Hund E, et al. First European consensus for diagnosis, management, and treatment of transthyretin familial amyloid polyneuropathy. Curr Opin Neurol 2016;29(Suppl 1):S14–26.
60. Ford ES, Giles WH, Dietz WH. Prevalence of the metabolic syndrome among US adults: findings from the third National Health and Nutrition Examination Survey. JAMA 2002;287(3):356–9.
61. Smith AG, Rose K, Singleton JR. Idiopathic neuropathy patients are at high risk for metabolic syndrome. J Neurol Sci 2008;273(1–2):25–8.
62. Tesfaye S, Chaturvedi N, Eaton SE, et al. Vascular risk factors and diabetic neuropathy. N Engl J Med 2005;352(4):341–50.
63. Look ARG. Effects of a long-term lifestyle modification programme on peripheral neuropathy in overweight or obese adults with type 2 diabetes: the Look AHEAD study. Diabetologia 2017;60(6):980–8.
64. Smith AG, Russell J, Feldman EL, et al. Lifestyle intervention for pre-diabetic neuropathy. Diabetes Care 2006;29(6):1294–9.
65. Brannagan TH 3rd, Hays AP, Chin SS, et al. Small-fiber neuropathy/neuronopathy associated with celiac disease: skin biopsy findings. Arch Neurol 2005;62(10):1574–8.
66. Hoitsma E, Faber CG, van Santen-Hoeufft M, et al. Improvement of small fiber neuropathy in a sarcoidosis patient after treatment with infliximab. Sarcoidosis Vasc Diffuse Lung Dis 2006;23(1):73–7.
67. Vinik AI, Strotmeyer ES, Nakave AA, et al. Diabetic neuropathy in older adults. Clin Geriatr Med 2008;24(3):407–35, v.
68. Acevedo JC, Amaya A, Casasola Ode L, et al. Guidelines for the diagnosis and management of neuropathic pain: consensus of a group of Latin American experts. J Pain Palliat Care Pharmacother 2009;23(3):261–81.
69. Bohlega S, Alsaadi T, Amir A, et al. Guidelines for the pharmacological treatment of peripheral neuropathic pain: expert panel recommendations for the middle East region. J Int Med Res 2010;38(2):295–317.

70. Bril V, England J, Franklin GM, et al. Evidence-based guideline: treatment of painful diabetic neuropathy: report of the American Academy of Neurology, the American Association of Neuromuscular and Electrodiagnostic Medicine, and the American Academy of Physical Medicine and Rehabilitation. Neurology 2011; 76(20):1758–65.

71. Dworkin RH, O'Connor AB, Audette J, et al. Recommendations for the pharmacological management of neuropathic pain: an overview and literature update. Mayo Clin Proc 2010;85(3 Suppl):S3–14.

72. Hovaguimian A, Gibbons CH. Diagnosis and treatment of pain in small-fiber neuropathy. Curr Pain Headache Rep 2011;15(3):193–200.

73. Moulin D, Boulanger A, Clark AJ, et al. Pharmacological management of chronic neuropathic pain: revised consensus statement from the Canadian Pain Society. Pain Res Manag 2014;19(6):328–35.

74. Gilron I, Bailey JM, Tu D, et al. Nortriptyline and gabapentin, alone and in combination for neuropathic pain: a double-blind, randomised controlled crossover trial. Lancet 2009;374(9697):1252–61.

75. Demant DT, Lund K, Finnerup NB, et al. Pain relief with lidocaine 5% patch in localized peripheral neuropathic pain in relation to pain phenotype: a randomised, double-blind, and placebo-controlled, phenotype panel study. Pain 2015;156(11):2234–44.

76. Finnerup NB, Attal N, Haroutounian S, et al. Pharmacotherapy for neuropathic pain in adults: a systematic review and meta-analysis. Lancet Neurol 2015; 14(2):162–73.

77. Hoffman EM, Watson JC, St Sauver J, et al. Association of long-term opioid therapy with functional status, adverse outcomes, and mortality among patients with polyneuropathy. JAMA Neurol 2017;74(7):773–9.

Cancer and Peripheral Nerve Disease

Jonathan Sarezky, MD, George Sachs, MD, PhD, Heinrich Elinzano, MD,
Kara Stavros, MD*

KEYWORDS

- Neuropathy • Chemotherapy • Paraneoplastic • Radiation • Plexopathy

KEY POINTS

- Cancer-related neuropathy may be caused by direct tumor invasion or compression of nerve structures, the effects of chemotherapy or immune checkpoint inhibitors, radiation, surgery, or paraneoplastic syndromes.
- The most common presentation of chemotherapy-induced peripheral neuropathy is a symmetric, stocking-glove distribution of predominantly sensory symptoms.
- Some chemotherapy can cause symptoms of neuropathy that may progress for several months after discontinuation of treatment, a phenomenon known as coasting.
- Chemotherapy-induced neuropathy is treated symptomatically but in some cases may involve dose reduction or change of chemotherapy agent.
- Paraneoplastic syndromes necessitate prompt initiation of immunomodulatory therapy.

INTRODUCTION

As the mortality associated with many forms of cancer improves, patients with cancer face disabling complications from both the disease and its treatments. Among these, peripheral neuropathy (PN) continues to be highly prevalent among patients with cancer. PN commonly results in symptoms of pain, numbness, and weakness that can be both unpleasant and debilitating. Neuropathy can affect patients at all stages of malignancy—it can be a presenting symptom, a side effect of therapy, or a lingering malady during remission. This review presents a summary of the clinical presentations and etiologies of PN associated with malignancy as well as current treatment strategies.

BACKGROUND

Chemotherapy-induced PN is the most common type of neuropathy seen in patients with cancer, with variable reports of incidence ranging from 19% to more than 85%.[1]

Alpert Medical School of Brown University, Rhode Island Hospital, 593 Eddy Street APC5, Providence, RI 02903, USA
* Corresponding author.
E-mail address: Kara_stavros1@brown.edu

Clin Geriatr Med 37 (2021) 289–300
https://doi.org/10.1016/j.cger.2021.01.003
0749-0690/21/© 2021 Elsevier Inc. All rights reserved.

In 1 meta-analysis examining more than 4000 patients receiving chemotherapy, the prevalence of PN was 68%.[1] Of these patients, 30% continued to report chronic symptoms of PN 6 months after therapy was completed. In addition to chemotherapy-induced PN, patients with cancer also may develop neuropathy related to radiation, immune checkpoint inhibitors, direct tumor involvement of nerve structures, or paraneoplastic syndromes, causing a wide range of symptoms. The incidence of these complications is less well studied.

The disability associated with cancer-related PN cannot be overstated. PN can cause severe distal numbness and pain (often difficult to control with analgesic medications), imbalance leading to falls, vision abnormalities, and pain in the pharynx or larynx, among other symptoms. As such, PN can result in significant impairments in quality of life, mobility, social life, and occupational duties. Studies of patients with chemotherapy-induced PN have demonstrated lower scores on measures of quality of life, physical functioning, and social functioning compared with patients without PN undergoing chemotherapy.[2,3] In addition, cancer-related PN may burden patients as well as the health care system as a whole financially; a large-scale review of insurance claims records between 1999 and 2006 showed that patients with a diagnosis of PN had an average of $17,344 greater health care costs than patients without PN.[4]

CAUSES AND CLINICAL PRESENTATIONS

Ascertaining the etiology of neuropathy in a patient with cancer is essential for determining the approach to treatment. In some cases, diagnosis of neuropathy may even be the first sign that leads to an initial diagnosis of cancer.

Neuropathy Induced by Anticancer Drugs

PN is a common, debilitating side effect of many chemotherapeutic agents (**Table 1**). PN can limit the dosing of chemotherapy and may continue to burden patients for years after it is discontinued. These drugs can induce PN through a variety of neurotoxic mechanisms that ultimately result in the induction of neuroinflammation and the altered excitability of peripheral neurons.[5]

Chemotherapy-induced PN first was implicated in the vinca alkaloids, in particular vincristine. Patients receiving this chemotherapy may develop a dose-dependent, predominantly sensory neuropathy manifested by numbness and painful paresthesias in the hands and feet. Autonomic neuropathy also is common, resulting in symptoms, such as paralytic ileus, orthostatic hypotension, and urinary dysfunction. Symptoms generally improve after cessation of the drug, although in some cases neuropathic symptoms can progress or even worsen.[6] In patients with certain hereditary neuropathies (such as Charcot-Marie-Tooth disease), vincristine can result in a fulminant onset of severe weakness and numbness in all extremities.[6,7] The rapidity of this presentation can mimic Guillain-Barré syndrome, and these medications should be avoided in these patients.

Platinum-based chemotherapies, including cisplatin, carboplatin, and oxaliplatin, also can cause PN. Cisplatin and carboplatin can cause a cumulative dose-dependent PN featuring distal sensory loss, painful paresthesias, and sensory ataxia (ie, imbalance resulting from impaired proprioception). Cisplatin-induced PN can exhibit a coasting phenomenon, in which the accumulation of the drug in dorsal root ganglia may result in the new presentation or continued worsening of neuropathy symptoms for several months after the drug has been stopped.[6] Oxaliplatin is notable in that it can cause both acute and chronic forms of PN. The acute form, which occurs in up to 90% of patients to varying degrees, causes pain and discomfort in the distal

Table 1
Overview of neuropathy symptoms associated with key anticancer drugs

Anticancer Drug	Clinical Features and Complications	Treatment
Vinca alkaloids (eg, vincristine)	• Distal predominant sensory and/or motor symptoms • Autonomic involvement (ileus, orthostatic hypotension, bladder dysfunction) • Cranial neuropathies may be seen	• Prognosis is variable and depends on the specific drug—often improves but may result in chronic persistent symptoms • Pharmacologic and nonpharmacologic symptom management
Taxanes (eg, paclitaxel)	• Distal predominant sensory symptoms • Motor or autonomic symptoms may occur	• Consider chemotherapy dose modification or cessation if treatment of early or severe symptoms.
Platinum compounds (eg, cisplatin, carboplatin, oxaliplatin)	• Distal predominant sensory symptoms • May exhibit a coasting phenomenon • Oxaliplatin may cause acute sensory symptoms shortly after initiation of infusion, often aggravated by cold	• Avoid use if possible in patients with hereditary neuropathy (Charcot-Marie-Tooth disease)
Thalidomide	• May present with sensory, motor, and/or autonomic symptoms	
Bortezomib	• Distal predominant sensory symptoms • Mild weakness or autonomic symptoms may also be see	
Suramin	• Sensory and/or motor symptoms	
Ixabepilone	• Sensory, motor, and/or autonomic symptoms may occur	
Immune checkpoint inhibitors (eg, ipilimumab)	• Length dependent polyneuropathy • Demyelinating polyneuropathy • Sensory neuronopathy • Myositis • Meningoradiculitis • Myasthenia gravis • Central nervous system complications	• Consider cessation of therapy if symptoms develop • Can respond to treatment with steroids or other immunotherapy

extremities, often triggered by cold.[8,9] This typically resolves within 1 week to 2 weeks, although often incompletely.[9] In addition to the acute form of PN, oxaliplatin causes a dose-dependent chronic PN, consisting of numbness and tingling in the distal extremities that may persist even after treatment. Like cisplatin, oxaliplatin also may exhibit a coasting phenomenon.

Taxanes, including paclitaxel, docetaxel, and cabazitaxel, are a third class of chemotherapy associated with a high prevalence of PN, estimated to be between 11% and 87%, with the highest rates seen in paclitaxel.[10] Sensation to all modalities can be affected, leading to distal numbness and tingling as well as loss of proprioception and balance. In some cases, weakness from motor neuropathy or autonomic dysfunction can occur.[6] Disabling PN symptoms have been reported up to 2 years after completing taxol therapy, ranging from mild to persistently severe.[11]

Other chemotherapeutic agents implicated in chemotherapy-induced PN are suramin, thalidomide, bortezomib, and ixabepilone, among others. Combinations of these agents or high single or cumulative doses may result in more severe presentations.

PN rarely has been associated with immune checkpoint inhibitors, occurring in less than 1% of treated patients.[12] This complication most commonly has been associated with ipilimumab and less so nivolumab or pembrolizumab, and PN related to immune checkpoint inhibitors tends to be more likely acute or subacute or non–length-dependent in pattern.[13] Cases of isolated cranial neuropathies and sensory neuronopathies have been reported as well.[13,14] Immune checkpoint inhibitors can induce autoimmunity, which has been implicated in many neurologic complications of these drugs affecting the peripheral nerves, muscles, neuromuscular junction, and central nervous system.[15] Guillain-Barré syndrome has been reported at a rate of 0.1% to 0.2%, with clinical and electrophysiological features typical of cases not associated with immune checkpoint inhibitors, although both albuminocytological dissociation and pleocytosis have been reported on cerebrospinal fluid studies.[14,16] Chronic inflammatory demyelinating polyneuropathy, meningoradiculitis, myositis, and myasthenia gravis also have been reported.[12,15] Providers should be acutely aware of these potential complications in patients receiving these medications and monitor closely for any new neurologic symptoms because these symptoms may progress rapidly.

Neuropathy Related to Direct Tumor Invasion

Cancer can cause neuropathy through direct invasion of the peripheral nervous system, although this is more rare than other cancer-associated mechanisms of neuropathy. Nerve roots and nerve plexuses tend to be more vulnerable to direct invasion, although this is variable based on the type of underlying malignancy.[17] Neurolymphomatosis is one example, encompassing neuropathies caused by the spread of different forms of leukemia and non-Hodgkin lymphoma.[18] The distribution of nerve involvement is variable and can include peripheral sensory or motor nerves, spinal nerves, the brachial or lumbosacral plexuses, or cranial nerves. Therefore, the presentation of neurolymphomatosis can be highly variable in individual patients. Solid tumor involvement of peripheral nerves also can occur, albeit less commonly. For example, rectal, cervical, and prostate cancers have been shown to invade nearby nerve structures.[19,20]

In the context of a known malignancy, a new focal neurologic deficit, in particular one that is not in the distribution of a common compression neuropathy, warrants investigation for spread of neoplastic disease to nerve structures. Neuropathic symptoms, such as sensory loss, pain, or weakness in the distribution of a nerve root or plexus, even occasionally may be the first presenting symptoms of a cancer. Specific neurologic syndromes that can point toward a malignancy diagnosis have been described. For example, a lesion to the submandibular branch of the trigeminal nerve, colloquially known as the numb chin syndrome, is highly associated with an underlying malignancy and metastatic disease.[21] Patients present with anesthesia to the lip or chin that usually is unilateral, although bilateral involvement can occur. In the absence of a known alternative cause, such a presentation should prompt a work-up for metastatic disease as well as consideration of additional studies, such as lumbar puncture.

Neuropathy Related to Paraneoplastic Syndromes

Paraneoplastic syndromes can cause multiple neurologic syndromes and may present even before the diagnosis of cancer. For the diagnosis of a neurologic paraneoplastic syndrome, the 2004 diagnostic criteria from the Paraneoplastic Neurological

Syndrome-European Consortium incorporated the presence of a classical paraneo-plastic neurologic syndrome, the presence of positive onconeural antibodies, the presence of a known malignancy, and response to immunotherapy.[22] Although not all criteria must be present for a diagnosis, various combinations of these criteria can lead to diagnoses of either definite or possible paraneoplastic neurologic syn-dromes. Recognition of classical paraneoplastic syndromes as well as a high index of suspicion in a patient with a known malignancy, therefore, will help clinicians diag-nose these conditions. Although some classical syndromes are discussed in this article, the diversity and variability of paraneoplastic neurologic syndromes must be emphasized.[23]

Sensory neuronopathy is one such classical paraneoplastic syndrome. A neuronop-athy (as opposed to a neuropathy) specifically involves damage to the cell body of the sensory neuron located in the dorsal root ganglion. Approximately 70% to 80% of all malignancy-associated cases of subacute sensory neuronopathy occur in the context of small cell lung cancer, most of which are associated with anti-Hu antibodies (anti-neuronal nuclear antibody type 1, anti-ANNA1),[24] although other malignancies and an-tibodies can be implicated in neuronopathies as well. Certain key clinical features can help differentiate a sensory neuronopathy from the more common axonal neuropathy. For example, symptoms often are asymmetric and can involve the upper extremities or proximal lower extremities, in contrast to the length-dependent pattern of a classic axonal PN. Proprioception often is affected, leading to prominent sensory ataxia and poor balance. The time course of a sensory neuronopathy is variable, ranging from subacute to even fulminant in some cases. Anti-Hu paraneoplastic syndromes typi-cally are associated with sensory neuronopathies, as described previously; however, less commonly, they may present with mixed sensorimotor, pure motor, or autonomic involvement. Another example to be familiar with is paraneoplastic syndromes asso-ciated with anti-CRMP5 (CV2). These antibodies often are associated with small cell lung cancer or a thymoma and can present with neuropathy, asymmetric painful rad-iculopathy, and even spinal cord involvement.[25] Cases of demyelinating polyneuropa-thies, such as Guillain-Barré syndrome and Chronic inflammatory demyelinating polyneuropathy, however, have been described in association with Hodgkin and non-Hodgkin lymphomas. Although these may represent a possible paraneoplastic syndrome, there have not been consistently identified associated onconeural antibodies.[26]

Monoclonal gammopathies, which are present in 3% to 4% of adults over age 50, also commonly feature associated neuropathy.[27] Please refer to Yaowaree Leavell and Susan C. Shin's article, "Paraproteinemias and Peripheral Nerve Disease"; and Stephen Cox and Kelly G. Gwathmey's article, "Chronic Immune-Mediated Poly-neuropathies," in this issue, for a more detailed discussion.

Neuropathy due to Iatrogenic Causes

Chemotherapy-induced PN, as described previously, is quite prevalent and disabling for certain drugs; however, other cancer treatments also may cause morbidity by damaging peripheral nerves. Cancer surgery can result in significant neuropathic pain. Neck surgeries, mastectomies, and thoracotomies all are procedures associated with a significant degree of neuropathic pain.[28] In postmastectomy pain syndrome, surgical trauma can result in injury to branches of the intercostal nerves or branches of the brachial plexus. Approximately half of respondents in 1 survey had some degree of mastectomy-related pain at a mean of 3.2 years postsurgery.[29] Patients typically present with numbness, paresthesias, or pain near the operative site, axilla, chest wall, or ipsilateral arm. Younger age, concomitant radiation or chemotherapy, and type of procedure may be risk factors for persistent pain, although the evidence is inconsistent.[30]

Neuropathy can develop in association with radiation therapy as well, often presenting in a delayed fashion months to years after radiation is completed. Prominent among radiation nerve injuries are radiation-induced plexopathies, both of the brachial plexus and lumbosacral plexus. The risk of neuropathy is dose-dependent; radiation-induced brachial plexopathy rates have been described at 66% when associated with higher doses of radiation used in the era before modern dosing but only 1% to 2% when associated with lower doses.[31] Radiation plexopathies typically present with sensory loss and weakness in a limb near where prior radiation occurred, and there may be characteristic signs of myokymia on electrophysiologic studies. Any history of radiation therapy, even remote history, is important in diagnosis, because radiation-induced plexopathies can present as late as decades after therapy is completed.[31] Pain is not a common symptom early in the course of the disease, so presence of pain should raise suspicion for direct tumor invasion and recurrence of malignancy rather than radiation injury.

Neuropathy from Noncancer Causes

Even in patients with known malignancies, common causes of neuropathy still should be considered always. When a malignancy-related cause of neuropathy is identified (such as chemotherapy), controlling other potentially coexisting causes may help prevent worsening of neuropathic symptoms.[32] For patients who present with distal symmetric polyneuropathy, American Academy of Neurology guidelines recommend testing at a minimum for diabetes mellitus (fasting blood sugar or hemoglobin A_{1c}), vitamin B_{12}, methylmalonic acid, and serum protein immunofixation.[33] Diabetes mellitus is the most common cause of polyneuropathy in the developed world, comprising one-third of cases.[33] Vitamin deficiencies, such as vitamin B_{12}, vitamin E, thiamine, copper, and pyridoxine, may be important causes of neuropathy, particularly in cancer patients with impaired vitamin absorption due to gastrointestinal pathology or surgeries. Long-term excessive alcohol use should be elicited on taking a history, because this can cause or worsen PNs and may have a direct neurotoxic effect.[32]

GENERAL PRINCIPLES OF DIAGNOSIS

Primary care providers encounter PN (also known as polyneuropathy) frequently and it is 1 of the top 5 reasons for neurologic referral.[32] Polyneuropathies most commonly are axonal and typically occur in a length-dependent fashion. Clinical features of cancer-related PN are indistinguishable from other distal PN. Patients first may experience numbness, paresthesias, burning, or pain in the feet as well as impaired balance. Symptoms can progress further up the legs and eventually involve the arms, creating a symmetric stocking-glove distribution. Sensory symptoms usually precede motor symptoms, although in more advanced cases distal muscle weakness and atrophy can be observed. Reflexes are depressed or absent. Autonomic symptoms may be overlooked and can include postural hypotension or tachycardia, gastroparesis, urinary or bowel dysfunction, or sexual dysfunction. The time course of symptom progression is variable.

Although many PNs present with this distal axonal pattern, others follow alternate patterns that can hint at their underlying etiology. Marked sensory deficit asymmetry with proximal limb involvement can indicate a sensory neuronopathy. A mononeuritis multiplex pattern occurs when there is evidence of damage to at least 2 separate nerves occurring in a progressive, stepwise pattern. Although classically associated with neuropathies in vasculitic and autoimmune diseases, mononeuritis multiplex may occur in direct multifocal tumor involvement, neurolymphomatosis, or certain paraneoplastic conditions.[17,24]

Diagnosis of neuropathy related to malignancy is individualized and dependent on each patient's history and examination. Careful neurologic examination helps localize the symptoms further, and a neurologic consultation should be considered if there is suspicion for peripheral nerve involvement. Common diagnostic tests that may help establish the diagnosis include nerve conduction studies and electromyography, laboratory studies, and focused imaging. Clinicians should have a low threshold to image the brain and spinal cord for patients who have cancer and neurologic symptoms, particularly if headaches, back pain, cranial nerve deficits, hyperreflexia, increased tone, or bowel or bladder symptoms are present. Cerebrospinal fluid analysis also may be helpful to evaluate for signs of inflammation and to exclude leptomeningeal metastasis. In cases of paraneoplastic syndrome suspected, testing for paraneoplastic antibodies is recommended. Because the clinical presentations of specific paraneoplastic antibodies can vary widely, testing with an antibody panel is recommended over testing single antibodies.[34] In general, neuropathy caused by chemotherapy should be considered a diagnosis of exclusion, and efforts should be made to rule out other possible causes of neuropathy when this is suspected.

Early diagnosis of peripheral nerve disorders in the setting of malignancy is important for faster initiation of treatment, prevention of further loss of function, and providing appropriate patient counseling. Delay in diagnosis of peripheral nerve complications from malignancy sometimes can occur in the setting of postsurgical immobilization, reduced activity, or sedation, all of which may obscure symptoms.[28]

HOW IS CANCER-RELATED NEUROPATHY TREATED?

The approach to treatment of cancer-related neuropathy depends on the type and cause of the neuropathy. The overall aim of treatment is to minimize symptoms, improve quality of life, and prevent loss of function.

For all patients, addressing the underlying cancer with appropriate treatment and counseling is paramount. Other general principles include both pharmacologic and nonpharmacologic treatments for neuropathic pain and providing other supportive care as appropriate. Supportive measures include physical therapy for gait training physical therapy for gait training, occupational therapy, fall prevention counseling, bracing/orthotics, behavior modifications, assistive devices such as a walker, exercise, and home safety modifications (**Box 1**).

Chemotherapy-Related Neuropathy Treatment

More specific strategies for the treatment and prevention of chemotherapy-induced PN have been studied extensively. Clinical risk factors that appear to confer an increased risk for developing neuropathy from chemotherapy include higher cumulative dose and increased number of treatments.[35] Baseline neuropathy also may portend a higher risk for developing neuropathy.[35]

In order to minimize the severity of chemotherapy-induced PN, 1 important intervention to consider is dose modification. Patients' neurologic symptoms should be recorded at baseline and then monitored closely throughout treatment. Dose reduction or even treatment discontinuation should be considered if patients develop severe symptoms or if symptoms develop early in the course of the treatment.[36] These decisions should be made carefully, however, with consideration of the effect on the underlying malignant process and in consultation with the oncology treatment team.

Box 1
Nonpharmacologic approaches to treatment of neuropathy associated with cancer

- Gait or exercise training
- Occupational therapy
- Fall prevention counseling
- Home safety evaluation
- Bracing or orthotics, as indicated
- Assistive devices, as indicated
- Foot care
- Behavior modifications

Numerous neuroprotective agents have been studied in chemotherapy-induced PN with the goal of blocking the noxious effects of chemotherapy, thereby limiting neuronal damage and promoting peripheral nerve regeneration.[37] There are some data to suggest a beneficial effect from exercise[38] but none to strongly support any medications or supplements as protective in the setting of chemotherapy-induced PN.[38,39] More research is needed to determine effective preventative measures. One challenge is that an ideal neuroprotective agent must not reduce the antineoplastic effect of the chemotherapy, promote tumor growth, or cause significant additional side effects.

Duloxetine is the only medication that has been shown to help reduce pain in patients with painful chemotherapy-induced PN in a randomized, placebo-controlled trial.[40] Empiric use of other agents used for neuropathic pain, however, is common practice and may be considered based on their use in other neuropathic pain syndromes. These agents include gabapentin, pregabalin, and tricyclic antidepressants as well as numerous nonpharmacologic approaches. For further details on therapeutic agents, see the Elizabeth J. Pedowitz and colleagues' article, "Management of Neuropathic Pain in the Geriatric Population," in this issue. Although these treatments may help with neuropathic pain in chemotherapy-induced PN, there currently are not any specific treatments available to improve symptoms of numbness.

Immune Checkpoint Inhibitor Neuropathy Treatment

Management of neuropathy caused by treatment with immune checkpoint inhibitors differs from management of neuropathy associated with other types of anti-cancer drugs. Here, management typically involves suspending treatment with the immune checkpoint inhibitor and initiating steroids as well as consideration of intravenous immunoglobulin and/or plasma exchange. Treatment duration should take into account the long half-life of immune checkpoint inhibitors and should be initiated early, because symptoms may be rapidly progressive.[41] Retrial of an immune checkpoint inhibitor after neurologic side effects may be possible in some cases; however, this requires a careful analysis of the risks versus benefits of doing so, with particular consideration of the risks of further exacerbation of the neurologic symptoms.[13,14] No clear guidelines exist on when or whether to reinitiate an immune checkpoint inhibitor in these select cases. For cases of Guillain-Barré syndrome associated with the use of immune checkpoint inhibitors, there is a potential role of the use of steroids based on limited case studies.[14,41] This is in contrast to Guillain-Barré syndrome not associated with immune checkpoint inhibitors, for which steroids are not used.

Paraneoplastic Syndrome Treatment

For a suspected paraneoplastic neuropathy, management generally consists of work-up for primary malignancy (if not already identified) and cancer treatment. Outcomes are better with earlier identification.[42] Prompt treatment should be initiated, particularly in patients who are rapidly declining.[34] Although strong evidence for the effective treatment of paraneoplastic neuropathies is scarce due to lack of data, immunomodulatory therapy may be considered both during and after cancer treatment. This may include intravenous immunoglobulin, steroids, plasma exchange, or rituximab, among others. Combinations of these treatments may also be used to improve symptoms and prevent further decline.

SUMMARY

The presentation of neuropathy related to underlying malignancy or the neurotoxic effects of cancer treatments is variable. Early recognition is important so steps can be taken to prevent progression and worsening of neurologic symptoms and disability. Currently, there are no interventions known to prevent chemotherapy or immune checkpoint inhibitor related neuropathy. Treatment depends on the type and cause of the neuropathy and typically consists of management of neuropathic pain and other supportive measures. In some circumstances, modification or discontinuation of anticancer treatment should be considered. More research is needed to determine how to best prevent these neurologic complications in patients with cancer.

CLINICS CARE POINTS

- Cancer can affect the peripheral nervous system in numerous ways; therefore, the clinical presentation may be variable. The most common pattern seen is sensory deficits in a stocking-glove distribution in the setting of chemotherapy.

- Clinicians should be aware of the neurotoxic effects of chemotherapy agents and immune checkpoint inhibitors. Patients receiving these treatments should be monitored closely because modifications in treatment or cessation of therapy may be indicated if significant symptoms develop.

- Some chemotherapy can cause symptoms of neuropathy that may progress for several months after discontinuation of treatment, a phenomenon known as coasting.

- Non–cancer-related causes of neuropathy always should be considered and investigated. Chemotherapy-induced PN is a diagnosis of exclusion.

- Paraneoplastic syndromes affecting the peripheral nervous system may include neuropathies and neuronopathies. The most common of these is associated with anti-Hu antibodies; however, a paraneoplastic antibody panel is recommended in most cases when a paraneoplastic syndrome is suspected.

- Radiation-induced plexopathy can have a delayed onset, with presentation of symptoms occurring years after the completion of treatment in some cases.

- Care for the patient with peripheral nervous system complications of cancer is multidisciplinary and may include a patient's primary care provider, oncologist, and neurologist.

DISCLOSURE

The authors have nothing to disclose.

REFERENCES

1. Seretny M, Currie GL, Sena ES, et al. Incidence, prevalence, and predictors of chemotherapy-induced peripheral neuropathy: a systematic review and meta-analysis. Pain 2014;155(12):2461–70.
2. Hsu HT, Wu LM, Lin PC, et al. Emotional distress and quality of life during folinic acid, fluorouracil, and oxaliplatin in colorectal cancer patients with and without chemotherapy-induced peripheral neuropathy: a cross-sectional study. Medicine (Baltimore) 2020;99(6):e19029.
3. Mols F, Beijers T, Vreugdenhil G, et al. Chemotherapy-induced peripheral neuropathy and its association with quality of life: a systematic review. Support Care Cancer 2014;22(8):2261–9.
4. Pike CT, Birnbaum HG, Muehlenbein CE, et al. Healthcare costs and workloss burden of patients with chemotherapy-associated peripheral neuropathy in breast, ovarian, head and neck, and nonsmall cell lung cancer. Chemother Res Pract 2012;2012:913848.
5. Zajaczkowska R, Kocot-Kepska M, Leppert W, et al. Mechanisms of chemotherapy-induced peripheral neuropathy. Int J Mol Sci 2019;20(6):1451.
6. Quasthoff S, Hartung HP. Chemotherapy-induced peripheral neuropathy. J Neurol 2002;249(1):9–17.
7. Graf WD, Chance PF, Lensch MW, et al. Severe vincristine neuropathy in Charcot-Marie-Tooth disease type 1A. Cancer 1996;77(7):1356–62.
8. Beijers AJ, Mols F, Vreugdenhil G. A systematic review on chronic oxaliplatin-induced peripheral neuropathy and the relation with oxaliplatin administration. Support Care Cancer 2014;22(7):1999–2007.
9. Pachman DR, Qin R, Seisler DK, et al. Clinical course of oxaliplatin-induced neuropathy: results from the randomized phase III Trial N08CB (Alliance). J Clin Oncol 2015;33(30):3416–22.
10. Banach M, Juranek JK, Zygulska AL. Chemotherapy-induced neuropathies-a growing problem for patients and health care providers. Brain Behav 2017; 7(1):e00558.
11. Hershman DL, Weimer LH, Wang A, et al. Association between patient reported outcomes and quantitative sensory tests for measuring long-term neurotoxicity in breast cancer survivors treated with adjuvant paclitaxel chemotherapy. Breast Cancer Res Treat 2011;125(3):767–74.
12. Hottinger AF. Neurologic complications of immune checkpoint inhibitors. Curr Opin Neurol 2016;29(6):806–12.
13. Dubey DDW, David WS, Amato AA, et al. Varied phenotypes and management of immune checkpoint inhibitor-associated neuropathies. Neurology 2019;93(11): e1093–103.
14. Kolb NA, Trevino CR, Waheed W, et al. Neuromuscular complications of immune checkpoint inhibitor therapy. Muscle Nerve 2018;58:10–22.
15. Cuzzubbo S, Javeri F, Tissier M, et al. Neurological adverse events associated with immune checkpoint inhibitors: review of the literature. Eur J Cancer 2017; 73:1–8.
16. Dalakas MC. Neurological complications of immune checkpoint inhibitors: what happens when you 'take the brakes off' the immune system. Ther Adv Neurol Disord 2018;11. 1756286418799864.
17. Grisold W, Briani C, Vass A. Malignant cell infiltration in the peripheral nervous system. Handb Clin Neurol 2013;115:685–712.

18. Grisariu S, Avni B, Batchelor TT, et al. Neurolymphomatosis: an international primary CNS lymphoma collaborative group report. Blood 2010;115(24):5005–11.
19. Capek S, Howe BM, Amrami KK, et al. Perineural spread of pelvic malignancies to the lumbosacral plexus and beyond: clinical and imaging patterns. Neurosurg Focus 2015;39(3):E14.
20. Capek S, Howe BM, Tracy JA, et al. Prostate cancer with perineural spread and dural extension causing bilateral lumbosacral plexopathy: case report. J Neurosurg 2015;122(4):778–83.
21. Ryba F, Rice S, Hutchison IL. Numb chin syndrome: an ominous clinical sign. Br Dent J 2010;208(7):283–5.
22. Graus F, Delattre JY, Antoine JC, et al. Recommended diagnostic criteria for paraneoplastic neurological syndromes. J Neurol Neurosurg Psychiatry 2004;75(8): 1135–40.
23. Lancaster E. Paraneoplastic disorders. Continuum (Minneap Minn) 2015;21(2): 452–75.
24. Antoine JC, Camdessanche JP. Paraneoplastic neuropathies. Curr Opin Neurol 2017;30(5):513–20.
25. Dubey D, Lennon VA, Gadoth A, et al. Autoimmune CRMP5 neuropathy phenotype and outcome defined from 105 cases. Neurology 2018;90(2):e103–10.
26. Rozlucka L, Semik-Grabarczyk E, Pietrukaniec M, et al. Demyelinating polyneuropathy and lymphoplasmacytic lymphoma coexisting in 36-year-old man: a case report. World J Clin Cases 2020;8(12):2566–73.
27. Chaudhry HM, Mauermann ML, Rajkumar SV. Monoclonal gammopathy-associated peripheral neuropathy: diagnosis and management. Mayo Clin Proc 2017;92(5):838–50.
28. Marchettini P, Formaglio F, Lacerenza M. Iatrogenic painful neuropathic complications of surgery in cancer. Acta Anaesthesiol Scand 2001;45(9):1090–4.
29. Belfer I, Schreiber KL, Shaffer JR, et al. Persistent postmastectomy pain in breast cancer survivors: analysis of clinical, demographic, and psychosocial factors. J Pain 2013;14(10):1185–95.
30. Jung BF, Ahrendt GM, Oaklander AL, et al. Neuropathic pain following breast cancer surgery: proposed classification and research update. Pain 2003; 104(1–2):1–13.
31. Delanian S, Lefaix JL, Pradat PF. Radiation-induced neuropathy in cancer survivors. Radiother Oncol 2012;105(3):273–82.
32. Watson JC, Dyck PJ. Peripheral neuropathy: a practical approach to diagnosis and symptom management. Mayo Clin Proc 2015;90(7):940–51.
33. Russell JA. General approach to peripheral nerve disorders. Continuum (Minneap Minn) 2017;23(5, Peripheral Nerve and Motor Neuron Disorders):1241–62.
34. Galli J, Greenlee J. Paraneoplastic diseases of the central nervous system. F1000Res 2020;9. F1000 Faculty Rev-167.
35. Li T, Timmins HC, Lazarus HM, et al. Peripheral neuropathy in hematologic malignancies - Past, present and future. Blood Rev 2020;43:100653.
36. Markman M. Chemotherapy-induced peripheral neuropathy: underreported and underappreciated. Curr Pain Headache Rep 2006;10(4):275–8.
37. Forman AD. Peripheral neuropathy and cancer. Curr Oncol Rep 2004;6(1):20–5.
38. Dorsey SG, Kleckner IR, Barton D, et al. The national cancer institute clinical trials planning meeting for prevention and treatment of chemotherapy-induced peripheral neuropathy. J Natl Cancer Inst 2019;111(6):531–7.
39. Hershman DL, Lacchetti C, Loprinzi CL. Prevention and management of chemotherapy-induced peripheral neuropathy in survivors of adult cancers:

American Society of Clinical Oncology Clinical Practice guideline summary. J Oncol Pract 2014;10(6):e421–4.

40. Smith EM, Pang H, Cirrincione C, et al. Effect of duloxetine on pain, function, and quality of life among patients with chemotherapy-induced painful peripheral neuropathy: a randomized clinical trial. JAMA 2013;309(13):1359–67.

41. Santomasso BD. Anticancer drugs and the nervous system. Continuum (Minneap Minn) 2020;26(3):732–64.

42. Koike H, Sobue G. Paraneoplastic neuropathy. Handb Clin Neurol 2013;115: 713–26.

Paraproteinemias and Peripheral Nerve Disease

Yaowaree Leavell, MD, Susan C. Shin, MD*

KEYWORDS

- Paraproteinemia • Peripheral nerve disease • Neuropathy • Amyloidosis

KEY POINTS

- All patients with new clinical or electrodiagnostic peripheral neuropathy should receive serologic screening for paraproteinemia (IFE, SPEP).
- CIDP, POEMS, an Multiple Myeloma are typically associated with IgG and IgA paraproteins while DADS and Waldenstrom's Macroglobulinemia are associated with IgM.
- Electrodiagnostic testing allows for more precise localization and classification of the neuropathy, differentiating between sensory vs motor, and axonal vs demyelinating processes.
- Severe autonomic dysfunction in the presence of rapidly progressive peripheral neuropathy is a hallmark of AL amyloidosis and hATTR and should prompt further testing.
- Recent advances in the diagnosis and treatment of hATTR include widely available low-cost serum and saliva genetic testing and two highly effective oligonucleotide agents.

INTRODUCTION

Paraproteinemias are a diverse group of diseases defined by the presence of a serum monoclonal protein (M-protein) due to aberrant overproduction by a monoclonal plasma cell population. Peripheral neuropathy (also known as polyneuropathy [PN]) can be the presenting symptom of a paraproteinemia. If a serum paraprotein is discovered, it then must be determined whether it is related to the neuropathy. With new disease-modifying treatments available, the ability to diagnose and treat paraprotein-associated PNs never has been more important. This article provides a clinical overview, diagnosis, and treatment of the major paraprotein-related PNs, including monoclonal gammopathy of undetermined significance (MGUS), multiple myeloma (MM), transthyretin amyloidosis (TTR), light chain (AL) amyloidosis, Waldenström macroglobulinemia (WM), and POEMS syndrome (**Table 1**).

MONOCLONAL GAMMOPATHY OF UNDETERMINED SIGNIFICANCE

MGUS is the most common and benign of the paraproteinemias, with a reported prevalence of 3.2% over age 50 and 5.3% over age 70.[1] Prevalence is higher among

Department of Neurology, Icahn School of Medicine at Mount Sinai, New York, NY, USA
* Corresponding author. 1468 Madison Avenue, New York, NY 10029.
E-mail address: susan.shin@mssm.edu

Clin Geriatr Med 37 (2021) 301–312
https://doi.org/10.1016/j.cger.2021.01.004
0749-0690/21/© 2021 Elsevier Inc. All rights reserved.

Table 1
Paraproteinemia-associated neuropathies: clinical and electrodiagnostic characteristics and treatment

	Paraprotein	Clinical Phenotype	Comments
MGUS	IgA or IgG	Phenotype is variable, including CIDP, distal sensorimotor PN, etc.	M-protein likely is incidental
	IgM	Most common: DADS PN	Patients 90% male, 7th to 9th decades. 50% of patients anti-MAG positive, no clear effect on treatment response
		Less common: heterogenous, can include axonal presentations	
WM	IgM	Most common: DADS PN	Approximately half of demyelinating WM-associated PNs have anti-MAG reactivity.
POEMS syndrome	Most commonly lambda-type IgG or IgA	Proximal and distal sensorimotor PN, subacute and progressive. Often very disabling, can result in wheelchair dependence	Serum VEGF levels elevated
MM			
Myeloma-related PN	IgG > IgA, abnormal FLC ratio	Distal sensory ± mild motor symptoms, painless, slowly progressive	If prominent autonomic symptoms, consider concurrent AL amyloid
Amyloidosis			
hATTR amyloid	No M-protein. TTR fibril deposition in tissues	Prominent distal sensory symptoms and early autonomic failure, rapid progression over months to a few years to include motor impairment and disability	Family history, red-flag symptom clusters, severe early CTS, unexplained heart failure, and treatment refractory CIDP. Early genetic testing recommended
wtTTR	No M-protein. TTR fibril deposition in tissues	Mild distal sensorimotor PN	PN less common than in hATTR/AL
AL amyloid	Most commonly lambda light chain	Distal sensorimotor PN with small fiber sensory loss followed by large fiber, prominent autonomic symptoms	Similar autonomic and systemic symptom profile to hATTR, higher incidence hemodynamic instability, advanced cardiomyopathy. specific signs include periorbital purpura and macroglossia

Abbreviations: CMAP, compound muscle action potential; CV, conduction velocity; TLI, terminal latency index.

patients with PN than in the general population, varying by center from 17% to 71%.[2,3] It is defined by a serum M-protein concentration of less than 3 g/dL; absence of anemia; bone lesions; hypercalcemia; and a bone marrow plasma cell concentration of less than 10%.[4] Once hematologic malignancy is ruled out, MGUS neuropathy can be stratified by phenotype and M-protein, as described later.

IgM Monoclonal Gammopathy of Undetermined Significance

Of the immunoglobulin classes, IgM has the strongest association with neuropathy.[5] The most common phenotype is a distal acquired demyelinating symmetric (DADS) neuropathy and predominantly affects men ages 50 to 80. Patients present with minimal distal weakness and sensory loss in the feet and later the hands and prominent gait ataxia due to sensory loss. The DADS with IgM protein patient has a markedly poorer response (20%–30%) to chronic inflammatory demyelinating polyradiculoneuropathy (CIDP) therapies, including plasmapheresis and intravenous immunoglobulin (IVIG), compared with the CIDP variant DADS without M-protein.[3,6]

Approximately 50% of DADS with M-protein patients demonstrate IgM recognition of myelin-associated glycoprotein (MAG).[7] Although it generally is accepted that anti-MAG proteins have a causative role in neuropathy, treatment response is not different from DADS with M-protein without anti-MAG proteins. Anti-MAG patients present heterogeneously, with as many as 17% of patients showing atypical clinical features that did not resemble DADS.[8,9] Although laboratory evidence suggests a high titer threshold for positivity (>10,000 units) more predictably identifies typical DADS with M-protein phenotype, no significant difference in the antibody titers between typical and atypical cases has been shown.[7,8] Of the 50% of DADS with M-protein patients whose serum does not react to MAG proteins, approximately 75% react to ganglioside antibodies.[10]

Treatment of IgM monoclonal gammopathy of undetermined significance neuropathies

There are scant high-quality data available on the treatment of this classically refractory PN. Given the older demographic, slow progression, pure sensory symptoms, and poor treatment response, patients with mild symptoms often are counseled that risks of therapy may not outweigh benefits. IVIG is reasonably safe and well-tolerated but has shown only small short-term benefit of doubtful clinical significance in this population.[11] If no response is noted within 3 months, it is unlikely to be of help. Inteferon alfa-2a has been trialed with variable results and no consistently demonstrated benefit, but in small nonrandomized settings (under 10 subjects) it has been shown to improve disease in 1 patient and improve postural stability in a small group of patients. Cyclophosphamide has been used with some individual successes but never has been used in a trial. Pulse-dose intravenous steroids as monotherapy have not shown clear efficacy and have had an unacceptably high rate of steroid psychosis.[11]

Rituximab has been used for the past 15 years in the anti-MAG population and is of probable benefit for a subset of patients despite failure to meet primary efficacy endpoints in 2 randomized controlled trials (RCTs).[12–14] A 2016 Cochrane review found a homogenous trend toward efficacy across the 2 small RCTs and several nonrandomized studies examined.[11] In 2017, a small nonrandomized study demonstrated a 56% improvement rate after 1 cycle and a 72% improvement rate after 2 cycles.[15]

IgA and IgG Monoclonal Gammopathy of Undetermined Significance

There is no strong evidence to demonstrate an association between IgA or IgG M-proteins and PN by direct or autoimmune mechanisms.[5] This is underscored by their variable presentations, including length-dependent sensorimotor axonal neuropathies or proximal and distal sensorimotor demyelinating neuropathy typical of CIDP.[2] Patients with IgA or IgG M-proteins should be worked-up to rule out POEMS syndrome and MM. Patients with a chronic demyelinating neuropathy and IgG or IgA MGUS are considered no different from CIDP patients without an M-protein and should receive appropriate first-line therapies for CIDP.[16,17]

WALDENSTRÖM MACROGLOBULINEMIA

WM is a rare, slowly progressive IgM-associated lymphoma typically affecting older men. Fewer than 1% of patients are under the age of 40.[2] Presenting symptoms include shortness of breath, epistaxis, blurred vision, and dizziness all of which are secondary to serum hyperviscosity.[5] Serum levels of IgM are not diagnostic criteria, but 1 series found high levels of IgM (>1830 mg/dL) and low hemoglobin (<12.6) to have good sensitivity and specificity for predicting WM.[18] Neuropathy is common, found in 20% to 50% of patients, with increasing prevalence as disease progresses.[19]

Both IgM-MGUS and WM PN present most often with a DADS clinical phenotype (symmetric, distal, and sensory-predominant); however, IgM-MGUS predominantly is demyelinating whereas nearly two-thirds of WM patients have an axonal neuropathy.[18,19] Of the 2, the axonal type is more likely to demonstrate clinical and etiologic heterogeneity, with 1 study reporting a variety of underlying etiologies, including AL amyloidosis, multifocal motor neuropathy (MMN), vasculitis, and tumor infiltration. Some of these patients were found to have motor symptoms and, in rare instances, a proximal and distal distribution of weakness inconsistent with the DADS phenotype.

By contrast, the demyelinating neuropathy presents more homogenously with distal paresthesias and more prominent distal sensory loss. Prior case series have demonstrated a 50% to 65% prevalence of anti-Mag reactivity among WM patients with a demyelinating phenotype.[19,20] Rituximab can be offered as monotherapy in patients with mild disease and associated PN, whereas advanced disease may require chemotherapy.[21] Short courses of plasma exchange (PLEX) are indicated in patients with hyperviscosity syndrome.[22]

POEMS SYNDROME

POEMS syndrome is a rare multisystem syndrome characterized by the findings it is named for, including PN, organomegaly, endocrinopathy, monoclonal gammopathy, and skin changes. Common findings include papilledema, thickened hyperpigmented skin, edema, organomegaly, sclerotic bone lesions, thrombocytosis, and pulmonary hypertension.[23] M-protein titers generally are in the normal or mildly elevated range, usually IgA or IgG, and almost always lambda-type. It typically is associated with osteosclerotic myeloma and age of onset is in the fifth or sixth decade, in contrast to MM, which peaks in the seventh or eighth decade.[2,5] Unlike the PN of MM, neuropathy is a defining feature of the syndrome to the extent that it is the only presenting symptom in 50% of patients.[24]

Most patients present with distal paresthesias and sensory neuropathy, which progress to include motor weakness with significant functional disability, such that some patients are wheelchair-bound or bedbound.[5] As the motor weakness progresses, it can cause proximal in addition to distal weakness. Nerve conduction studies (NCSs) and electromyography (EMG) show significant diffuse demyelination and axonal loss.[25] The combination of proximal and distal weakness with subacute sensorimotor neuropathy and conduction slowing on EMG often leads to a misdiagnosis of CIDP. CIDP features of patchy demyelination, including temporal dispersion and conduction block, are absent.[25] Distal pain is more common and severe than with lower greater than upper limb involvement.[24] In addition to electrodiagnostic testing, screening low-resolution body CT with bone windows or PET or PET/computed tomography (CT) is suggested to look for organomegaly and bone lesions.[23]

Treatment entails treating the underlying disease while minimizing iatrogenic neurologic worsening. POEMS neuropathy does not respond to IVIG or PLEX. Patients with localized disease are recommended to receive radiotherapy only; neurologic treatment response begins approximately 6 months after radiotherapy with maximal benefit at 2 years to 3 years.[13] Patients receiving autologous stem cell transplant (ASCT) and chemotherapy have shown significant functional neurologic improvement.[14,26]

MULTIPLE MYELOMA

MM is defined by 10% or more plasma cells on a bone marrow study with serum or urine M-protein and evidence of renal dysfunction, anemia, hypercalcemia, or bone lesions.[5] PN has been reported in 7% to 54% of patients, depending on criteria used for diagnosis.[27]

Myeloma-related PN is mechanistically poorly understood. It presents as a slowly progressive, painless, axonal sensorimotor, sensory, or motor distal PN with absent ankle jerks and mild distal weakness and numbness. Although autonomic symptoms are uncommon, during their disease course approximately 10% to 15% of patients can develop AL amyloidosis (discussed later). Any patient with myeloma-related PN who develops significant autonomic symptoms should be evaluated for AL amyloidosis.[28] Treatment of myeloma-related PN involves therapy for the underlying disease as well as adequate neuropathic pain control and physical therapy.[5]

DIAGNOSTIC TESTING IN NONAMYLOID PARAPROTEINEMIC NEUROPATHIES
Serology and Blood Work

Diagnostic work-up for new-onset PN by history and examination should include screening for M-proteins and end-organ manifestations of disease. Other than TTR amyloidosis, all the disorders described in this article are defined by the presence of an M-protein. Serum protein electrophoresis (SPEP) offers quantification of protein level but is insensitive for serum protein less than 0.3 g/dL to 0.5 g/dL and cannot differentiate immunoglobulin type. Sensitivity is 87% for MM but as low as 50% to 66% for light chain deposition disease.[29] Serum immunofixation (IFE) offers a lower serum protein detection threshold (0.1 g/dL) and higher sensitivity across paraproteinemic disorders and can determine the immunoglobulin type. Free light chain assays offer 10 times the sensitivity of IFE, in the range of 82% to 88%. Serum and urine IFE with free light chain assays offers a 98% sensitivity for detecting an M-protein. Urine testing should include a 24-hour total urine collection for total protein. Given the high prevalence of multisystem disease in these disorders, blood counts and renal and liver function testing are recommended. Serologic testing for common treatable causes of neuropathy, including vitamin B_{12} and glucose intolerance, should be considered. If POEMS syndrome is suspected, serum vascular endothelial growth factor (VEGF) should be checked because levels greater than 1000 pg/mL have been found 100% sensitive and 92% specific in patients with M-protein and characteristic neuropathy.[14]

Nerve Conduction Studies and Electromyography

NCS/EMG testing should be performed to determine whether the phenotype is predominantly axonal or demyelinating and to rule out nonparaproteinemic disorders.

The combination of M-protein type and electrophysiologic profile should be taken into consideration to determine whether further serologic testing or invasive diagnostic procedures, including lumbar puncture and nerve or skin biopsy, are warranted.

Invasive Diagnostic Procedures

Nerve biopsy has become increasingly rare but can be considered for refractory chronic demyelinating disease or other clinical and electrophysiologic phenotypes, such as rapidly progressive axonal PNs. Pathology can provide information about inflammatory infiltrates, protein deposition, and other features of autoimmune, vasculitic, or neoplastic neuropathies. Therapy aimed at reducing the paraprotein level likely is not justified without biopsy-confirmed endoneurial paraprotein deposit, nerve reactivity to the paraprotein, or nerve cellular paraprotein infiltrates. In rare cases, pathologic confirmation of the M-protein in the nerve tissue has prompted aggressive immunotherapy, but there is scant evidence to support or refute this practice.[2,30] Lumbar puncture can be considered in any demyelinating neuropathy to demonstrate albuminocytologic dissociation but is of particular importance in patients with malignancy to rule out myelomatous involvement of the leptomeninges. Skin biopsy is performed when electrodiagnostic testing is normal and pure small fiber neuropathy is suspected.

AMYLOIDOSIS

Neuropathy is a common presenting symptom of amyloid disease. The mechanism of peripheral nerve injury is deposition of amyloid in various components of the nervous tissue, resulting in compression of the myelin sheath, disruption of the blood-nerve barrier, direct Schwann cell injury, and damage to the blood vessels supplying the nerve.[31] This article focuses on TTR amyloidosis and AL amyloidosis, which are distinct from the cerebral β-amyloidosis seen in Alzheimer dementia. Amyloid disease is discussed separately from the other paraproteinemias due to its unique clinical features and different diagnostic approach, attributed largely to the presence of both hereditary and acquired forms of amyloidosis.

Transthyretin Amyloidosis

TTR results from either excessive accumulation of normal transthyretin protein fibrils (wild-type TTR [wtTTR]) or from an autosomal dominant mutation in the transthyretin protein (hereditary amyloid TTR [hATTR]). Abnormal fibril deposition in various tissue sites results in organ dysfunction and structural disease.

Wild-type transthyretin amyloidosis

wtTTR, also referred to as senile amyloidosis, constitutes 48% of US TTR cases but only 5% of cases worldwide. Post mortem studies demonstrate the presence of TTR in up to 25% of the population over age 80 and is more common in men.[32]

Cardiomyopathy and arrhythmia are the predominant clinical manifestations of wtTTR. Patients present most commonly with exercise intolerance, which tends to progressively worsen over the course of a few years. Neuromuscular manifestations include lumbar spinal stenosis, carpal tunnel syndrome (CTS) (33%), and spontaneous biceps tendon rupture (33%).[33] Extracardiac manifestations, including peripheral (10%–12%) and autonomic neuropathy, are uncommon.[34,35]

Hereditary transthyretin amyloidosis

The clinical manifestations of hATTR are diverse and vary by mutation and region. They may be endemic, meaning localized with clear family history and early-onset disease, or nonendemic, meaning scattered with frequently negative family history and late-onset disease. Unlike wtTTR, the hereditary amyloidosis have frequent extracardiac manifestations, including prominent peripheral and autonomic neuropathy and end-organ damage (**Table 2**). Autonomic dysfunction is present in 75% of patients with hATTR, causing a range of gastrointestinal (GI) and sexual symptoms.[36] Patients require regular serum and urine screening for renal dysfunction and proteinuria. One notable early neurologic sign is CTS, which often is bilateral and precedes systemic symptoms by 7 years to 10 years.[37] In the authors' own practice, a high index of suspicion is maintained in young patients with severe CTS in a nondominant hand unexplained by occupation and a concerning family history.

Classically, hATTR PN presents as a small fiber sensory neuropathy causing allodynia, painful burning and tingling in the feet, and a length-dependent loss of pinprick sensation on examination.[31,35] This progresses over months to a few years to involve large sensory fibers, causing loss of vibration and position sense and gait instability with significant functional impairment. During later stages, motor fibers become involved, resulting in distal clinical weakness, which advances proximally within 4

Table 2
Red-flag symptom clusters in light chain and hereditary amyloid transthyretin amyloidosis

Organ System	Symptom	Associated Diagnostic Testing
Central nervous system	Headache, stroke-like episodes, progressive dementia	MRI brain, including with SWI or GRE sequence. Biopsy of leptomeninges and parenchyma (rare)
Ocular	Vitreous opacification, glaucoma, pupil abnormalities (scalloped, asymmetric)	Pupil examination, direct ophthalmoscopy, intraocular pressure testing
Renal	Proteinuria, renal failure	24 h urine protein, urine Bence Jones proteins, BMP, biopsy (rare)
Cardiovascular	Conduction block, arrhythmia, cardiomyopathy	EKG, echocardiogram, cardiac MRI, nuclear scintigraphy, endocardial biopsy, BNP, GFR, NT-proBNP, GD-15[a]
GI	Nausea, early satiety, diarrhea and constipation, weight loss. Organomegaly[a]	Clinical history, abdominal CT or ultrasound
Autonomic nervous system	Sexual dysfunction, sweating abnormalities, orthostatic hypotension, urinary retention	Quantitative sudomotor testing, tilt-table testing, postvoid residual
Peripheral nervous system	CTS (5–7 y before hATTR diagnosis). Distal paresthesias, numbness, gait unsteadiness. Progresses to include distal weakness, eventually also in hands and proximal limbs	Clinical examination, NCS/EMG. If CTS surgery, tenosynovium sample can be stained for congo red. Nerve biopsy (rare). Skin biopsy (small fiber neuropathy)
Other[a]	Macroglossia, periorbital purpura	Clinical examination

Abbreviations: BMP, basic metabolic panel; BNP, brain natriuretic peptide; EKG, electrocardiogram; GD-15, growth determination factor 15; GFR, glomerular filtration rate; GRE, gradient-recalled echo; MRI, magnetic resonance imaging; NT-proBNP, N-terminal pro-BNP; SWI, susceptibility-weighted imaging.
[a] More suggestive of AL amyloidosis.

years to 5 years of onset. NCS/EMG classically reveals an axonal distal sensorimotor neuropathy.[35]

There are several notable specific mutations in hATTR worth mentioning because they have specific phenotypes and demographics. Patients with the Val30Met mutation from the endemic regions including Sweden, Japan, Mallorca, Cyprus, and Portugal present with early-onset PN in the third or fourth decade. The disease course follows the typical pattern with prominent dysautonomia and red-flag symptom clusters, as described previously, and a clear family history of early progressive neuropathy. Patients from nonendemic regions present with a male-predominant late-onset form in the fifth decade; autonomic symptoms are less common; and progression is slower.[31,34] The most common mutation in the United States, Val122Ile, is best known as a late-onset heart failure variant, but rates of neuropathy still are as high as 10% to 38% in this population. Thr60Ala, the second most common variant in the United States, originating in Northern Ireland, has a mixed cardiac and neurologic phenotype, with high rates of CTS (70%) and PN in the fourth decade. Other rarer variants include Tyr77Ser, which presents with a rapidly progressive ataxia with diffuse areflexia and large fiber sensory loss, and Ala24Thr, which causes a pure motor weakness without sensory or autonomic features. Leu58Arg, Try114His, and Ile84Ser present with isolated CTS as the only neurologic manifestation.[31,34]

Light Chain Amyloidosis

AL amyloidosis is a multisystem disease most commonly affecting the kidneys, heart, GI tract, liver, and autonomic nervous system.[29] Renal involvement is prominent and cardiomyopathy occurs in 40% to 60% of patients, with more rapid progression than in TTR amyloid. Other symptoms specific to AL amyloidosis include waxy skin and skin nodules, periorbital purpura, macroglossia, coagulopathy, easy bruising, and lymphadenopathy.[38]

AL amyloid fibrils are formed from light chains secreted by an abnormal clonal plasma cell, or rarely clonal B-cell, population. Most AL amyloid patients have MGUS at the time of diagnosis, with approximately 10% to 15% developing comorbid MM.[29,35,38] Other rare etiologies of AL amyloid are WM and non-Hodgkin lymphoma. It is the most common form of amyloidosis in the United States, with a prevalence of 2.5 per 100,000.[31]

PN occurs in 17% to 35% of patients and often is found at the time of diagnosis; the average time from diagnosis to death for patients who present with PN is approximately 25 months to 35 months. Mortality is due most commonly to congestive heart failure or renal failure. Progression and pattern of neuropathy is similar to TTR amyloidosis, as described previously.[38] Unlike TTR PN, which presents with primarily sensory deficits, AL can present with mixed sensorimotor deficits approximately half of the time.[31]

Diagnostic Testing in Amyloid Neuropathy

For both TTR amyloidosis and AL amyloidosis, diagnosis hinges on identifying the fibril type, scope, and extent of organ involvement. Given that CTS precedes systemic TTR symptoms by 5 years to 7 years, it also is important to attend to the combination of CTS and red-flag symptom clusters. A compelling family history should trigger prompt genetic TTR testing, but it is important to remember than nonendemic genetic variants frequently have occurred in patients without a family history of disease.[39] Amyloid neuropathy should be considered in cases of rapidly progressive neuropathy, which are refractory to treatment.

Electrodiagnostic testing
Once amyloid PN is suspected clinically, initial work-up should include NCS/EMG to confirm and quantify neurologic involvement. The classic electrodiagnostic findings initially are an axonal-predominant distal sensorimotor neuropathy with distal denervation. Varying degrees of demyelination and slowing may be present, contributing to potential misdiagnosis of CIDP.[40]

Serology
Initial serum work-up for suspected amyloid PN should include IFE and SPEP to screen for M-proteins as well as kappa:lambda light chain ratio. M-proteins are expected to be absent in the TTR amyloidosis and present in AL amyloid, MGUS, WM, POEMS syndrome, and MM. In practice, however, M-proteins may be encountered even in TTR amyloid patients either as an incidental finding or an indicator that another disease process is present. Complete blood cell count, liver function, renal function, and creatine kinase should be checked to screen for myopathy and organ dysfunction.

Genetic testing
Genetic testing is the test of choice for hATTR amyloidosis. It largely has replaced the need for nerve biopsy given wide availability, affordability, and sensitivity of 99% for detection of pathogenic variants.[31] If there already is a known mutation identified in a patient's family member, it is reasonable to test selectively. Otherwise, sequencing of the entire TTR gene is recommended. If a genetic specialist is available in the region, the patient should be referred for testing and genetic counseling. Testing availability varies by region and can be obtained at low cost or no cost from some companies using mail-in serum or saliva samples.

Biopsy
Tissue confirmation of amyloid deposition by demonstrating green birefringence after Congo red staining remains the gold standard for diagnosis. This confirms the presence of amyloid fibrils but does not distinguish between fibril types. Common locations for biopsy are the subcutaneous fat pad, rectal mucosa, labial mucosa, salivary glands, kidneys, endocardium, and synovial samples sent from carpal tunnel surgery.[31,39] Lower-risk sites with reasonable yield, such as the fat pad, rectal, and labial mucosa, should be tried first.[35] Patients with autonomic or small fiber symptoms and normal EMG should be worked-up with skin biopsy. In addition to quantifying nerve fiber density to make a diagnosis of small fiber neuropathy, skin biopsy also can identify amyloid deposition in nerve fibers.[41]

Treatment of Transthyretin Amyloidosis Amyloid Neuropathy

Liver transplantation
Liver transplantation historically has been the gold standard for treatment of hATTR amyloidosis for eligible patients because this removes the site of mutant TTR synthesis. Benefit varies somewhat by mutation. Liver transplant does not stop the production of wtTTR.[31]

Pharmacotherapy
Pharmaceutical treatment modalities are classified by where they act along the TTR fibril formation pathway. Current approved therapies fall into 2 classes: fibril stabilizers and mRNA silencers. The latter are approved only for treatment of hATTR-related PN despite some evidence of cardiac benefit.[34]

Fibril stabilizers. Tafamidis is an oral agent that binds selectively to thyroxine-binding site of the TTR protein and prevents fibril aggregation and thus reduces tissue deposition.

A 2012 randomized placebo-controlled trial demonstrated delayed and reduced neurologic dysfunction and improved nutritional status in Val30Met patients with PN. A 2018 trial in patients with hATTR cardiomyopathy demonstrated lower mortality rates in 2.5 years and reduced decline in cardiac function scores. Tafamidis recently was approved by the Food and Drug Administration (FDA) for treatment of both wtTTR and hATTR cardiomyopathy. It has been used off-label for treatment of TTR neuropathy.

Diflunisal is a nonsteroidal anti-inflammatory agent that has been shown to have some efficacy as a fibril stabilizer via binding to the thyroxine-binding site of the TTR protein. Although it is not FDA-approved, several open-label nonrandomized trials have shown cardiac efficacy similar to tafamidis and 1 trial has shown reduction in neurologic impairment in hATTR patients. Diflunisal has been used off-label for both wtTTR and haTTR patients with either cardiomyopathy or neuropathy.

mRNA silencers. In 2018, 2 mRNA silencing agents, patisaran and inotersen, obtained FDA approval for the treatment of PN in hATTR in adults. Both agents act upstream at the transcription level to inhibit production of TTR protein tetramers before they can be assembled. The treatments likely not only slow the progression of neuropathy but also even may lead to dramatic improvements in neurologic status.

Treatment of Neuropathy in Light Chain Amyloidosis

The treatment of underlying AL amyloidosis may improve the associated neuropathy.[31] There are no specific therapies for PN related to AL amyloidosis. Available therapies for AL amyloidosis include ASCT with melphalan chemotherapy; cyclophosphamide, bortezomib, and dexamethasone in combination; leflunomide; and pomalidomide.[29,31]

SUMMARY

In conclusion, paraproteinemias are a diverse group of diseases that have frequent overlap and have a high association with serious forms of PN. Work-up for any patient with new-onset PN should include serologic and clinical screening for paraproteinemic disorders to avoid missing these potentially serious underlying causes. NCS/EMG may be needed to determine localization and guide treatment decisions. As the diagnostic and therapeutic landscape continues to evolve, interdisciplinary collaboration will be essential for optimal care in these complex patients.

CLINICS CARE POINTS

- CIDP with IgA or IgG MGUS is no different from classic CIDP without paraproteinemia and should receive appropriate first-line treatment.
- DADS PN with IgM M-protein is a distinct entity from DADS without M-protein (a CIDP variant) with poor treatment response to typical therapy; there is weak evidence in favor of rituximab.
- POEMS syndrome should be considered in new-onset demyelinating PN with IgG or IgA, skin changes, organomegaly, endocrinopathies, or bone lesions; serum VEGF levels greater than 1000 pg/ml are highly sensitive and specific in such patients.
- Amyloid neuropathy may mimic CIDP and should be considered in patients with refractory chronic demyelinating neuropathies.
- Available therapies for hATTR amyloid neuropathy include mRNA silencers (patisaran and inotersen) and the fibril stabilizers.

REFERENCES

1. Kyle RA, Therneau TM, Rajkumar SV, et al. Prevalence of monoclonal gammopathy of undetermined significance. N Engl J Med 2006;354(13):1362–9.
2. Raheja D, Specht C, Simmons Z. Paraproteinemic neuropathies. Muscle Nerve 2015;51(1):1–13.
3. Ramchandren S, Lewis RA. An update on monoclonal gammopathy and neuropathy. Curr Neurol Neurosci Rep 2012;12(1):102–10.
4. Kyle RA, Larson DR, Therneau TM, et al. Long-term follow-up of monoclonal gammopathy of undetermined significance. N Engl J Med 2018;378(3):241–9.
5. Mauermann ML. Paraproteinemic neuropathies. Continuum (Minneap Minn) 2014;20(5 Peripheral Nervous System Disorders):1307–22.
6. Saperstein DS, Katz JS, Amato AA, et al. Clinical spectrum of chronic acquired demyelinating polyneuropathies. Muscle Nerve 2001;24(3):311–24.
7. Pascual-Goñi E, Martín-Aguilar L, Lleixà C, et al. Clinical and laboratory features of anti-MAG neuropathy without monoclonal gammopathy. Sci Rep 2019;9(1): 6155.
8. Svahn J, Petiot P, Antoine JC, et al. Anti-MAG antibodies in 202 patients: clinicopathological and therapeutic features. J Neurol Neurosurg Psychiatry 2018;89(5): 499–505.
9. Campagnolo M, Ferrari S, Dalla Torre C, et al. Polyneuropathy with anti-sulfatide and anti-MAG antibodies: clinical, neurophysiological, pathological features and response to treatment. J Neuroimmunol 2015;281:1–4.
10. Dalakas MC. Advances in the diagnosis, immunopathogenesis and therapies of IgM-anti-MAG antibody-mediated neuropathies. Ther Adv Neurol Disord 2018; 11. 1756285617746640.
11. Lunn MP, Nobile-Orazio E. Immunotherapy for IgM anti-myelin-associated glycoprotein paraprotein-associated peripheral neuropathies. Cochrane Database Syst Rev 2016;(10):CD002827.
12. Léger JM, Viala K, Nicolas G, et al. Placebo-controlled trial of rituximab in IgM anti-myelin-associated glycoprotein neuropathy. Neurology 2013;80(24): 2217–25.
13. Nobile-Orazio E, Bianco M, Nozza A. Advances in the treatment of paraproteinemic neuropathy. Curr Treat Options Neurol 2017;19(12):43.
14. Lunn MP. Neuropathies and paraproteins. Curr Opin Neurol 2019;32(5):658–65.
15. Campagnolo M, Zambello R, Nobile-Orazio E, et al. IgM MGUS and Waldenstrom-associated anti-MAG neuropathies display similar response to rituximab therapy. J Neurol Neurosurg Psychiatry 2017;88(12):1094–7.
16. Latov N. Diagnosis and treatment of chronic acquired demyelinating polyneuropathies. Nat Rev Neurol 2014;10(8):435–46.
17. Stork AC, Lunn MP, Nobile-Orazio E, et al. Treatment for IgG and IgA paraproteinaemic neuropathy. Cochrane Database Syst Rev 2015;(3):CD005376.
18. Klein CJ, Moon JS, Mauermann ML, et al. The neuropathies of Waldenström's macroglobulinemia (WM) and IgM-MGUS. Can J Neurol Sci 2011;38(2):289–95.
19. Viala K, Stojkovic T, Doncker AV, et al. Heterogeneous spectrum of neuropathies in Waldenström's macroglobulinemia: a diagnostic strategy to optimize their management. J Peripher Nerv Syst 2012;17(1):90–101.
20. Levine T, Pestronk A, Florence J, et al. Peripheral neuropathies in Waldenström's macroglobulinaemia. J Neurol Neurosurg Psychiatry 2006;77(2):224–8.

21. Kapoor P, Ansell SM, Fonseca R, et al. Diagnosis and management of waldenström macroglobulinemia: mayo stratification of macroglobulinemia and risk-adapted therapy (mSMART) Guidelines 2016. JAMA Oncol 2017;3(9):1257–65.

22. Rosenbaum E, Marks D, Raza S. Diagnosis and management of neuropathies associated with plasma cell dyscrasias. Hematol Oncol 2018;36(1):3–14.

23. Dispenzieri A, Kourelis T, Buadi F. POEMS syndrome: diagnosis and investigative work-up. Hematol Oncol Clin North Am 2018;32(1):119–39.

24. Nasu S, Misawa S, Sekiguchi Y, et al. Different neurological and physiological profiles in POEMS syndrome and chronic inflammatory demyelinating polyneuropathy. J Neurol Neurosurg Psychiatry 2012;83(5):476–9.

25. Mauermann ML, Sorenson EJ, Dispenzieri A, et al. Uniform demyelination and more severe axonal loss distinguish POEMS syndrome from CIDP. J Neurol Neurosurg Psychiatry 2012;83(5):480–6.

26. Karam C, Klein CJ, Dispenzieri A, et al. Polyneuropathy improvement following autologous stem cell transplantation for POEMS syndrome. Neurology 2015; 84(19):1981–7.

27. Morawska M, Grzasko N, Kostyra M, et al. Therapy-related peripheral neuropathy in multiple myeloma patients. Hematol Oncol 2015;33(4):113–9.

28. Rutten KHG, Raymakers RAP, Minnema MC. 'Transformation' from amyloid light chain amyloidosis to symptomatic multiple myeloma. Neth J Med 2018;76(5): 249–50.

29. Ryšavá R. AL amyloidosis: advances in diagnostics and treatment. Nephrol Dial Transplant 2019;34(9):1460–6.

30. Vallat JM, Magy L, Sindou P, et al. IgG neuropathy: an immunoelectron microscopic study. J Neuropathol Exp Neurol 2005;64(5):386–90.

31. Kaku M, Berk JL. Neuropathy associated with systemic amyloidosis. Semin Neurol 2019;39(5):578–88.

32. Brunjes DL, Castano A, Clemons A, et al. Transthyretin cardiac amyloidosis in older Americans. J Card Fail 2016;22(12):996–1003.

33. Galant NJ, Westermark P, Higaki JN, et al. Transthyretin amyloidosis: an under-recognized neuropathy and cardiomyopathy. Clin Sci (Lond) 2017;131(5): 395–409.

34. Ruberg FL, Grogan M, Hanna M, et al. Transthyretin amyloid cardiomyopathy: JACC state-of-the-art review. J Am Coll Cardiol 2019;73(22):2872–91.

35. Wechalekar AD, Gillmore JD, Hawkins PN. Systemic amyloidosis. Lancet 2016; 387(10038):2641–54.

36. Conceição I, González-Duarte A, Obici L, et al. Red-flag" symptom clusters in transthyretin familial amyloid polyneuropathy. J Peripher Nerv Syst 2016; 21(1):5–9.

37. Karam C, Dimitrova D, Christ M, et al. Carpal tunnel syndrome and associated symptoms as first manifestation of hATTR amyloidosis. Neurol Clin Pract 2019; 9(4):309–13.

38. Hazenberg BP. Amyloidosis: a clinical overview. Rheum Dis Clin North Am 2013; 39(2):323–45.

39. Finsterer J, Iglseder S, Wanschitz J, et al. Hereditary transthyretin-related amyloidosis. Acta Neurol Scand 2019;139(2):92–105.

40. Cortese A, Vegezzi E, Lozza A, et al. Diagnostic challenges in hereditary transthyretin amyloidosis with polyneuropathy: avoiding misdiagnosis of a treatable hereditary neuropathy. J Neurol Neurosurg Psychiatry 2017;88(5):457–8.

41. Kapoor M, Rossor AM, Jaunmuktane Z, et al. Diagnosis of amyloid neuropathy. Pract Neurol 2019;19(3):250–8.

Guillain-Barré Syndrome and Other Acute Polyneuropathies

Justin Kwan, MD[a],*, Suur Biliciler, MD[b]

KEYWORDS

- Guillain-Barré syndrome • Diagnosis • Therapy • Disease management
- Dysautonomia • Aged

KEY POINTS

- Guillain-Barré syndrome (GBS) is an acute monophasic autoimmune neuropathy frequently preceded by respiratory or gastrointestinal infections, and the most common subtypes are acute inflammatory demyelinating polyradiculoneuropathy, acute motor axonal neuropathy, and Miller Fisher syndrome.
- GBS is a clinical diagnosis and diagnostic studies are useful to exclude GBS mimics and to characterize the neuropathy.
- Older patients are at increased risk for respiratory and cardiovascular complications associated with GBS and require close clinical monitoring.
- A multidisciplinary approach to treatment of motor impairment, pain, and fatigue is recommended in GBS patients.

INTRODUCTION

Guillain-Barré syndrome (GBS) is the most common cause of acute neuropathy, characterized by rapidly progressive weakness affecting the extremity and cranial muscles.[1] It is a heterogeneous disorder, with patients having varying degrees and severity of motor, sensory, and autonomic dysfunction, and recognized clinical variants, including acute inflammatory demyelinating polyradiculoneuropathy (AIDP), acute motor axonal neuropathy (AMAN), and Miller Fisher syndrome.[1,2] Current evidence suggests that GBS is caused by an aberrant autoimmune response to a stimulation of the immune system, such as an infection.[3] Despite the many advances in the understanding of the pathophysiology of GBS, a diagnosis relies mainly on clinical

[a] National Institute of Neurological Disorders and Stroke, National Institutes of Health, Building 10, Room 1D45, MSC 1140, 10 Center Drive, Bethesda, MD 20814, USA; [b] Department of Neurology, The University of Texas Health Science Center at Houston, McGovern Medical School, 6431 Fannin Street MSE#466, Houston, TX 77030, USA
* Corresponding author.
E-mail address: justin.kwan@nih.gov

Clin Geriatr Med 37 (2021) 313–326
https://doi.org/10.1016/j.cger.2021.01.005
0749-0690/21/Published by Elsevier Inc.

geriatric.theclinics.com

findings of progressive weakness and areflexia.[4] These core clinical features are remarkably similar to the historic reports of GBS, including that by Landry, who in 1859, described 10 patients with acute ascending or generalized paralysis.[5] The 1916 descriptions by Guillain, Barré, and Strohl of a syndrome of progressive weakness, sensory abnormalities, diminished deep tendon reflexes, and albumincytological dissociation (elevated protein and normal cell count) in the cerebrospinal fluid (CSF) in 2 French soldiers included all major features of GBS.[6,7] This review discusses the clinical features, diagnosis, treatment, and pathophysiology of GBS.

EPIDEMIOLOGY AND RISK FACTORS

GBS is a rare disorder and the incidence is approximately 0.81 to 1.89 cases per 100,000 person-years in Europe and North America, although there are some geographic variations worldwide.[8,9] Men have a higher risk than women, and there appears to be an age-related increase in risk up to the ninth decade of life, with a 20% increase in incidence for every 10 years increase in age.[8,10] In approximately two-thirds of patients, the symptoms of GBS are preceded by an infection within the prior 4 weeks. The most common is a diarrheal illness caused by *Campylobacter jejuni*.[11] In the elderly, the preceding illness may be shorter in duration and may be more likely to be a flulike syndrome rather than a gastrointestinal disorder.[12] There are other infectious organisms associated with GBS, including human immunodeficiency virus (HIV), cytomegalovirus, Epstein-Barr virus, influenza A virus and influenza B virus, and, more recently the Zika virus.[11,13,14] The severe acute respiratory syndrome (SARS)–coronavirus 2 (SARS–CoV-2), which had infected more than 23 million people worldwide as of August 2020, raised concerns that there may be an increase in the number of GBS worldwide.[15] A recent review of the neurologic complications of SARS–CoV-2 showed that GBS infrequently occurs in COVID-19 patients, although long-term close surveillance for GBS cases remains necessary.[16]

Vaccination, surgery, anesthesia, trauma, and use of recreational drugs also are reported to be associated with GBS.[1,17] A frequent patient concern is the risk for GBS after influenza vaccination because of the association between GBS and the H1N1 influenza A vaccination in 1976 and 2009.[18,19] Epidemiologic studies of the relationship between influenza vaccination and GBS suggest that vaccine related GBS is rare.[20,21] Recurrent GBS also is not observed in patients who previously were diagnosed with GBS and subsequently received influenza vaccinations.[22,23] Furthermore, the potential risk for developing GBS after influenza infections may be greater than the risk for developing GBS after influenza vaccination.[21,24] For these reasons, clinicians should follow the Centers for Disease Control and Prevention guidelines when counseling patients about the risks and benefits of seasonal influenza vaccination.[25] The basis for the association between GBS and surgery is uncertain. A recent study suggests that autoimmune disorders and malignancies may be more common in patients who develop GBS after surgical procedures.[26] Any proposed mechanism based on these findings is speculative; however, the study does bring to attention the importance of considering GBS as a diagnosis in individuals who have acute postoperative weakness and a known history of autoimmune disease or malignancy.

CLINICAL FEATURES

In AIDP, the most common subtype of GBS, the earliest symptoms consist of abnormal sensation, such as tingling or numbness in the toes or fingers, followed by limb weakness.[1,2] Pain symptoms, such as sciatica; muscle pain involving the trunk, low back, or leg muscles; neck stiffness; and uncomfortable paresthesia, can be prominent and severe, and may persist for several months after the acute phase of the disorder.[27–30] In a substantial number of patients, pain symptoms even may precede the onset of muscle weakness by up to 2 weeks.[30] Although the sensory symptoms tend to precede the motor symptoms in AIDP, weakness is the predominant finding on examination. The most common pattern of weakness is that of ascending paralysis, starting in the distal legs up to the thighs, followed by upper limb and cranial muscles.[1,7] Bulbar and respiratory muscles frequently are affected. In some patients, muscle weakness may be more prominent in the proximal muscles (ie, shoulder and hip girdle muscles), and rarely is the weakness confined only to the lower extremities.[31,32] Nearly all patients have diminished or absent deep tendon reflexes on neurologic examination.[33]

Autonomic dysfunction is a common and important clinical feature of GBS requiring vigilant monitoring because of the associated increase in morbidity and mortality.[34] Although sinus tachycardia is the most common abnormality, labile blood pressure and cardiac tachyarrhythmia can occur, requiring cardiac monitoring in the intensive care unit.[34] Pupillary, gastrointestinal, or urinary dysfunction or pandysautonomia also can occur.[35] Autonomic dysfunction may be more common in GBS patients who develop respiratory failure and is independently associated with the need for mechanical ventilation.[36] It is important to systemically assess symptoms of autonomic dysfunction so that medical interventions can be initiated early.

Acute Clinical Course

In most GBS patients, progressive motor weakness occurs over the course of 1 week to 3 weeks, and nearly all patients have maximum weakness by 4 weeks.[33,37] Rarely does weakness continue to worsen beyond 4 weeks or 5 weeks, and when it does, an alternate diagnosis should be considered.[33] Although the severity of symptoms in GBS can vary widely between patients, most GBS patients require close observation in the hospital because of the potential risk for life-threatening complications, such as respiratory failure. Older patients, in particular, tend to progress to maximum weakness over a shorter duration and more often have severe disease symptoms resulting in complete loss of independent ambulation, respiratory failure, or death.[10,12] Preexisting comorbidities and increased frequency of severe disease in older GBS patients necessitate more intensive clinical monitoring and symptomatic management to decrease risk for infections, thromboembolism, and decubitus ulcers.

In the course of GBS, approximately half of the patients have facial weakness and swallowing difficulty, which can cause malnutrition or dehydration and increase the possibility for aspiration.[1] Bulbar muscle weakness may be more common in older patients whereas facial weakness occurs less often.[10,12] One-third of patients have respiratory failure and require ventilatory support in the intensive care unit.[1,33] Because cranial and respiratory muscles function frequently are impaired, and may occur within the first week of symptom onset or during treatment, it is prudent to evaluate the respiratory status and swallowing function in GBS patients closely until the nadir of the weakness is reached.[31,38] The most consistent clinical features predictive of impending respiratory failure and need for mechanical ventilation are short duration from symptom onset to hospital admission (less than 7 days), severe limb muscle weakness, and facial and bulbar muscle weakness.[36,38,39]

Guillain-Barré Syndrome Variants

GBS is a heterogeneous disorder consisting of a few different subtypes unified by the shared feature that the cause is an autoimmune injury of the peripheral nerves (**Box 1**).[40] Although the terms GBS and AIDP frequently are used interchangeably,

---

Box 1
Guillain-Barré syndrome subtypes

AIDP

AMAN

Acute motor and sensory axonal neuropathy

Miller Fisher syndrome

Acute autonomic neuropathy

Bickerstaff brainstem encephalitis

GBS represents a spectrum of autoimmune neuropathies in which AIDP is the most common subtype. In AIDP, patients have symptoms of motor and sensory nerve dysfunction and dysautonomia.[1] The presence of a demyelinating neuropathy is determined by findings on nerve conduction studies.[1,41] In AMAN, unlike in AIDP, patients have motor symptoms and do not have sensory abnormalities.[40] Miller Fisher syndrome is a rare subtype of GBS in which the patients have the classic triad of ophthalmoplegia, ataxia, and areflexia.[42,43]

GUILLAIN-BARRÉ SYNDROME DIAGNOSIS

A diagnosis of GBS should be suspected in any patient who presents with an acute onset of progressive weakness. GBS is a clinical diagnosis. In the diagnostic criteria developed by the National Institute of Neurological and Communicative Disorders and Stroke (now the National Institute of Neurological Disorders and Stroke [NINDS]), the only features required for diagnosis are cranial, truncal, and/or limb muscle weakness and diminished or loss of deep tendon reflexes.[4,37] There are clinical features that do not support a diagnosis of GBS (**Box 2**), and, when present, should prompt the clinician to consider an alternate diagnosis. There is no 1 single diagnostic test that is specific for GBS; however, diagnostic studies are useful to exclude GBS mimics and characterize the neuropathy. Although a diagnosis of GBS may be relatively straightforward in patients who have the characteristic history and findings on examination, the correct diagnosis may be missed in patients early in the disease course when the main symptoms are sensory abnormalities or pain. An important differential

---

Box 2
Neurologic features inconsistent with diagnosis of Guillain-Barré syndrome

Progressive or relapsing weakness beyond 8 weeks

Truncal sensory level

Hyperreflexia[a] and pathologic reflexes (clonus or extensor plantar response)

Persistent asymmetric weakness

Prominent sensory symptoms without weakness

Bowel and bladder sphincter dysfunction at symptom onset

Severe respiratory dysfunction with preserved limb strength

[a] Rarely, the deep tendon reflexes can be hyperactive in the presence of anti-GD1a antibodies.

---

diagnosis to consider in patients who have progressing ascending paralysis is a spinal cord disorder. In contrast to patients with spinal cord disorders who tend to have a sensory level, hyperactive deep tendon reflexes below the cord lesion, and pathologic reflexes, such as Babinski sign, GBS patients have distal (ie, in the hands and feet) sensory abnormalities and hypoactive or absent deep tendon reflexes on examination. Spine imaging with magnetic resonance imaging should be performed in patients with possible spinal cord disorders.

The most helpful diagnostic studies to obtain when evaluating patients suspected of having GBS are CSF studies and electrophysiologic testing consisting of nerve conduction studies and electromyography.[2] Although these diagnostic tests are not required to diagnose GBS, they can be supportive of a diagnosis if the results show the typical abnormalities. The original CSF findings of increased protein and normal cell count, also known as albumin-cytological dissociation, described by Guillain, Barré, and Strohl in 1916, continue to be recognized as the characteristic CSF profile.[6,44] In most GBS patients, the CSF white blood cell count is less than 5 cells/μL, and cell count greater than 50 cells/μL should raise suspicion for an alternate diagnosis, such as infection or malignancy.[33,45] GBS can be the initial presentation of HIV infection, and HIV testing should be considered in patients who have CSF pleocytosis.[46] Importantly, the absence of elevated CSF protein should not dissuade a clinician from diagnosing GBS, especially when the test is obtained very early after symptom onset.[1] The CSF protein can be normal in up to half of GBS patients within the first week.[33,47] Elevated CSF protein in isolation is not diagnostic of GBS nor is it predictive of disease severity. A modest increase in CSF protein is nonspecific and can be seen in other neurologic and non-neurological disorders.[48–50] The finding of albumin-cytological dissociation to support a GBS diagnosis requires appropriate clinical context.

Nerve conduction studies and electromyography are electrophysiologic studies that are used to evaluate the integrity of the peripheral nervous system. These studies can support GBS diagnosis, determine GBS subtypes, prognosticate outcome, and exclude GBS mimics.[33,45] Although electrophysiologic studies can assist in diagnosing GBS and its variants, these tests may not be readily available in all hospitals due to the requirement for highly trained personnel and specialized equipment. Therefore, initiating treatment of GBS should not be delayed because of an inability to obtain these studies. Electrophysiologic studies can distinguish AIDP from AMAN. In AIDP, the nerve conduction studies show findings of a demyelinating neuropathy affecting motor and sensory nerves, whereas in AMAN, the nerve conduction studies show findings of an axonal neuropathy only affecting the motor nerves.[41,51] It may be helpful to distinguish AIDP from AMAN because some studies suggest a more favorable prognosis in AIDP compared with AMAN, although this is not a consistent finding.[52–55] There are some limitations to electrophysiologic testing. Nerve conduction studies can be normal or show minor nonspecific abnormalities in GBS patients during the first week after symptom onset.[41,54] Additionally, the study may not be able to determine the GBS subtype early in the disease course.[33] If an electrophysiologic study is performed within the first week of symptom onset and is nondiagnostic, repeat testing in 1 week to 2 weeks can be considered.

Routine laboratory studies do not contribute to diagnosing GBS, but they are helpful to exclude other causes of peripheral neuropathy that mimic GBS, such as infection, malignancy, or other autoimmune disorders.[56] Because neoplastic disorders are much more common in the elderly, it is important to consider and evaluate for a neoplastic or paraneoplastic cause of neuropathic symptoms in older patients.[57] Serum ganglioside antibody testing is not helpful in most GBS patients; however, testing for anti-GQ1b IgG antibody should be considered in Miller Fisher syndrome, especially if there is diagnostic uncertainty.[43,58] Fecal testing and serology to detect C jejuni infection or serology to evaluate for infection by Epstein-Barr virus or cytomegalovirus can be obtained, but these studies do not contribute to GBS diagnosis and are not helpful in determining the clinical subtype or prognosis.[3] A complete blood cell count; electrolytes panel; glucose, renal, and liver function studies; and coagulation profile often are obtained to evaluate for other medical disorders and to monitor for side effects due to GBS treatments. Serial serum electrolyte panels are recommended in all GBS patients because hyponatremia secondary to syndrome of inappropriate secretion of antidiuretic hormone (SIADH) can be seen in up to half of all patients.[59,60] Older patients may be more vulnerable to this complication because of age-related loss of water regulation mechanisms and a predisposition to developing SIADH. Furthermore, older patients frequently have disorders requiring use of medications in which hyponatremia is a known side effect.[61]

PATHOPHYSIOLOGY

Pathologic studies of peripheral nerves from GBS patients provided the earliest evidence that GBS may be an inflammatory disorder.[62] The pathology was present in the nerve roots, nerve trunks, and distal nerve branches. The abnormalities on nerve biopsy included myelin and axonal destruction and infiltration by mononuclear cells and macrophages.[1,63] Subsequent studies showed that T cells and B cells, macrophages, and complement activation contributed to peripheral nerve injury in GBS.[1,3,31] The potential immune mechanism was clarified further by studies demonstrating an association between a preceding infection and GBS. The finding that respiratory and gastrointestinal infections by C jejuni, cytomegalovirus, and Epstein-Barr virus were associated with GBS led to the hypothesis that GBS may be a postinfectious immune-mediated disorder.[11,64] It is postulated that the epitopes on the surface of pathogens mimic components of the peripheral nerve ganglioside, triggering an aberrant activation of the immune system. In susceptible individuals, these events cause an autoimmune injury of the peripheral nerve myelin sheath and axons.[1,3,9]

GUILLAIN-BARRÉ SYNDROME MANAGEMENT
Acute Treatment

Treatment of GBS requires a multidisciplinary approach. On admission to the hospital, all GBS patients should be observed in an intermediate monitoring unit or in the intensive care unit. Serial pulmonary function tests, including forced vital capacity, maximum inspiratory pressure, and/or maximum expiratory pressure, are essential to evaluate for impending respiratory failure. These measures should be performed every 1 hours to 4 hours, depending on a patient's clinical status. Frequent blood pressure and heart rate measurements are necessary to evaluate for autonomic dysfunction, especially cardiovascular dysregulation, which can be present in approximately two-thirds of patients.[65] When stable, patients can be transferred to a medical unit with telemetry monitoring.

Intravenous immunoglobulin (IVIG) and plasma exchange are both effective in GBS, especially if IVIG is given within the first 2 weeks and plasma exchange is given within the first 4 weeks of disease onset.[66–68] There are no data suggesting that 1 treatment is superior to the other.[69] The choice of therapy should be based on the availability of IVIG or plasma exchange as well as the clinical characteristics of each patient.

IVIG can be administered 0.4 g/kg daily for 5 days or 1 g/kg daily for 2 days. The most common side effects include are headaches, aseptic meningitis, nausea, and electrolyte abnormalities, such as hypocalcemia. Hemolytic anemia, renal dysfunction, and thrombotic events, such as deep vein thrombosis, pulmonary embolus, acute coronary syndrome, and cerebral ischemia, are among the possible complications. There may be an increased risk for serious complications in older patients receiving IVIG. Special attention should be given to the IVIG concentration and other solution additives and adequate hydration prior to IVIG infusions. Older patients require close clinical and laboratory monitoring for side effects during treatment and posttreatment.[70] Corticosteroid as a monotherapy is not effective in GBS.[71] Corticosteroids may be useful if aseptic meningitis develops as a side effect of IVIG.

In GBS, plasma exchange frequently is administered in 5 to 7 sessions over a course of 1 week to 2 weeks.[67] Plasma exchange combined with IVIG or corticosteroids does not provide better outcomes.[66,72] Administering plasma exchange immediately after IVIG may worsen the outcome because it risks removal of IVIG. Moreover, it is not considered cost effective.[73] Side effects of plasma exchange consist of, but are not limited to, allergic reaction, hypotension, hypocalcemia, and filter clotting. In addition, plasma exchange carries risks related to central catheter placement including infection, bleeding, and pneumothorax.[74] There are few data on the safety of plasma exchange in older patients. Because other medical comorbidities are more common in older GBS patients, the risk for complication related to plasma exchange likely is increased.[10,75,76]

During the acute hospitalization, all GBS patients should be engaged in physical and occupational therapy as early as possible to minimize complications related to prolonged immobility, such as deconditioning. Inpatient rehabilitation may be considered in the appropriate patient. Physical exercise is associated with long-term improved health outcomes in GBS patients. Cycling appears to be the most effective form of exercise.[77] A cautious approach to physical activity should be taken to avoid over exercise that can lead to extreme fatigue.[78] The long-term prevalence of health-related quality of life determinants, such as fatigue, pain, and depression, in GBS patients is not completely known.[79] Clinicians should be alert to these symptoms in the acute setting because of the impact on patient participation during rehabilitation. Pain symptoms should be treated aggressively, and gabapentin is suggested as the first-line treatment of choice for neuropathic pain.[80] Fatigue symptoms can be responsive to physical therapy, exercise, and cognitive behavioral therapy.[81]

Recurrent Guillain-Barré Syndrome and Treatment-Related Fluctuations

Typically, GBS is a monophasic disorder, and recurrent GBS is uncommon, occurring in approximately 5% to 6% of patients.[82–84] Among patients who have recurrent GBS, most patients have 1 recurrence and it is rare for a patient to have more than 2 recurrences.[83] Infection is the most common antecedent event prior to GBS recurrence and the interval between recurrence can range from months to many years.[83,84] Because of the rarity of recurrent GBS, a diagnosis of chronic inflammatory demyelinating polyneuropathy (CIDP) should be considered in patients whose symptoms continue to worsen beyond 8 weeks or who have relapses within a few months after an episode of GBS. Like GBS, CIDP is an autoimmune demyelinating polyradiculoneuropathy, and the clinical symptoms and findings are similar to GBS.[85] In approximately 16% of CIDP patients, the initial neuropathic symptoms can be rapidly progressive within 4 weeks and may be difficult to distinguish from GBS.[86] The distinction, however, is important because CIDP is a chronic neuropathy with a relapsing course, and CIDP can respond to corticosteroid therapy unlike GBS.[87] Recurrent GBS and CIDP also should be distinguished from treatment-related fluctuations (TRFs), which is a worsening in GBS symptoms after an initial improvement or stabilization following treatment with IVIG or plasma exchange.[88] TRFs typically occur within a few days after a patient has completed a course of therapy and can be seen in up to 10% of GBS patients.[88–90] Some patients may have 2 episodes of TRFs and in rare patients a third episode can occur.[89,90] Nearly all TRFs occur within 8 weeks from GBS symptom onset, and if a patient has another relapse past this time frame or has more than 3 relapses, a diagnosis of CIDP should be considered.[90,91] In most patients, the relapsing symptoms due to TRFs respond to another course of IVIG or plasma exchange.[88,89] The cause of TRFs is unknown. One hypothesis is that the duration of the treatment effect is shorter than the disease activity, and the immune modulating effect of the therapy dissipates before the autoimmune process resolves.[88]

Prognosis and Long-Term Symptoms

All patients gradually improve over weeks to months, with most improvement in motor function occurring during the first year.[92] A majority of patients can walk independently within 6 months from the time of symptom onset even in patients who required mechanical ventilation, but the time to recovery in older patients may be slower.[2,10,92] Although prognosis tend to be favorable overall, the mortality rate in GBS continues to range from 3% to 6% despite improvements in care in the intensive care setting.[93,94]

Early mobilization with physical and occupational therapy as early as possible is important to minimize complications related to prolonged immobility, such as deconditioning. Inpatient rehabilitation may be considered in the appropriate patient. Physical exercise after acute hospitalization is associated with long-term improved health outcomes in GBS patients. Cycling appears to be the most effective form of exercise.[77] A cautious approach to physical activity should be taken to avoid over exercise that can lead to extreme fatigue.[78]

In addition to motor impairment, many GBS patients have persistent symptoms of pain, fatigue, and mood disorders.[1,95,96] The long-term prevalence of these health-related quality of life determinants in GBS patients is not completely known.[79] Fatigue may be unrelated to persistent motor impairment or the severity of weakness during the acute phase of the GBS.[22,97,98] In these patients, a structured exercise program may be beneficial.[99,100] Chronic pain is another significant source of morbidity. Severe muscular, neuropathic, or joint pain can be present in up to one-third of patients.[22,30,98] Because GBS patients may experience several pain symptoms concurrently caused by different mechanisms, a multidisciplinary approach should be taken to treat the pain syndrome. Although physical therapy may improve pain, many patients require chronic neuropathic pain medications.[101] Depression and/or anxiety triggered by the acute paralytic disorder is not infrequent and may be exacerbated by pain.[22,102] In patients who have symptoms of depression and anxiety, referral to mental health care providers for psychosocial support or to psychiatry for pharmacologic treatment should be considered. Medications with dual effectiveness for both psychiatric and neuropathic pain symptoms should be considered in order to minimize polypharmacy in older patients.

SUMMARY

GBS is a complex autoimmune disorder that can affect multiple organ systems and cause persistent impairment, having an impact on an individual's functional independence. A correct diagnosis leading to early treatments and appropriate interventions can mitigate the risk for poor outcome in geriatric patients diagnosed with GBS.

CLINICS CARE POINTS

- Autonomic dysfunction is common in GBS and it is important to screen for symptoms of dysautonomia.
- Risk factors for respiratory insufficiency requiring mechanical ventilation include duration from symptom onset to hospitalization, facial and/or bulbar weakness, and severity of limb weakness.
- Bedside pulmonary function testing is recommended to screen for impending respiratory failure.
- Normal CSF protein does not exclude a diagnosis of GBS.
- An alternate diagnosis, such as an acute HIV infection, should be considered if there is CSF pleocytosis, especially when more than 50 cells/μL are present.
- IVIG and plasma exchange both are effective treatments of GBS.
- Corticosteroid is not an effective treatment of GBS.
- Sequential use of IVIG and plasma exchange is not recommended.

ACKNOWLEDGMENTS

This work was supported in part by the Intramural Research Program of the NIH, NINDS.

DISCLOSURE

The authors have nothing to disclose.

REFERENCES

1. Ropper AH. The Guillain-Barré syndrome. N Engl J Med 1992;326(17):1130–6.
2. Leonhard SE, Mandarakas MR, Gondim FAA, et al. Diagnosis and management of Guillain-Barré syndrome in ten steps. Nat Rev Neurol 2019;15(11):671–83.
3. Yuki N, Hartung HP. Guillain-Barré syndrome. N Engl J Med 2012;366(24): 2294–304.
4. Asbury AK, Arnason BGW, Karp HR, et al. Criteria for diagnosis of Guillain-Barré syndrome. Ann Neurol 1978;3(6):565–6.
5. Pearce JM. Octave Landry's ascending paralysis and the Landry-Guillain-Barre-Strohl syndrome. J Neurol Neurosurg Psychiatry 1997;62(5):495–500.
6. Guillain G, Barré JA, Strohl A. [Radiculoneuritis syndrome with hyperalbuminosis of cerebrospinal fluid without cellular reaction. Notes on clinical features and graphs of tendon reflexes. 1916]. Ann Med Interne (Paris) 1999;150(1):24–32.
7. Hughes RAC, Cornblath DR, Willison HJ. Guillain-barré syndrome in the 100 years since its description by Guillain, Barré and Strohl. Brain 2016;139(11): 3041–7.
8. Sejvar JJ, Baughman AL, Wise M, et al. Population incidence of Guillain-Barré syndrome: a systematic review and meta-analysis. Neuroepidemiology 2011; 36(2):123–33.
9. van den Berg B, Walgaard C, Drenthen J, et al. Guillain-Barré syndrome: pathogenesis, diagnosis, treatment and prognosis. Nat Rev Neurol 2014;10(8): 469–82.
10. Peric S, Berisavac I, Stojiljkovic Tamas O, et al. Guillain-Barré syndrome in the elderly. J Peripher Nerv Syst 2016;21(2):105–10.

11. Jacobs BC, Rothbarth PH, van der Meché FG, et al. The spectrum of antecedent infections in Guillain-Barré syndrome: a case-control study. Neurology 1998;51(4):1110–5.

12. Sridharan GV, Tallis RC, Gautam PC. Guillain-Barré syndrome in the elderly. A retrospective comparative study. Gerontology 1993;39(3):170–5.

13. Hao Y, Wang W, Jacobs BC, et al. Antecedent infections in Guillain-Barré syndrome: a single-center, prospective study. Ann Clin Transl Neurol 2019;6(12): 2510–7.

14. Leonhard SE, Conde RM, de Assis Aquino Gondim F, et al. Diagnosis and treatment of Guillain-Barré syndrome during the Zika virus epidemic in Brazil: a national survey study. J Peripher Nerv Syst 2019;24(4):340–7.

15. Bigaut K, Mallaret M, Baloglu S, et al. Guillain-Barré syndrome related to SARS-CoV-2 infection. Neurol Neuroimmunol Neuroinflamm 2020;7(5):e785.

16. Romero-Sánchez CM, Díaz-Maroto I, Fernández-Díaz E, et al. Neurologic manifestations in hospitalized patients with COVID-19: the ALBACOVID registry. Neurology 2020;95(8):e1060–70.

17. Tan IL, Ng T, Vucic S. Severe Guillain-Barré syndrome following head trauma. J Clin Neurosci 2010;17(11):1452–4.

18. Schonberger LB, Bregman DJ, Sullivan-Bolyai JZ, et al. Guillain-barre syndrome following vaccination in the national influenza immunization program, United States, 1976–1977. Am J Epidemiol 1979;110(2):105–23.

19. Wise ME, Viray M, Sejvar JJ, et al. Guillain-Barre syndrome during the 2009-2010 H1N1 influenza vaccination campaign: population-based surveillance among 45 million Americans. Am J Epidemiol 2012;175(11):1110–9.

20. Vellozzi C, Broder KR, Haber P, et al. Adverse events following influenza A (H1N1) 2009 monovalent vaccines reported to the vaccine adverse event reporting system, United States, October 1, 2009-January 31, 2010. Vaccine 2010;28(45):7248–55.

21. Lehmann HC, Hartung HP, Kieseier BC, et al. Guillain-Barré syndrome after exposure to influenza virus. Lancet Infect Dis 2010;10(9):643–51.

22. Kuitwaard K, Bos-Eyssen ME, Blomkwist-Markens PH, et al. Recurrences, vaccinations and long-term symptoms in GBS and CIDP. J Peripher Nerv Syst 2009; 14(4):310–5.

23. Baxter R, Lewis N, Bakshi N, et al. Recurrent Guillain-Barre syndrome following vaccination. Clin Infect Dis 2012;54(6):800–4.

24. Poland GA, Jacobsen SJ. Influenza vaccine, Guillain-Barré syndrome, and chasing zero. Vaccine 2012;30(40):5801–3.

25. Prevention CfDCa. Seasonal influenza vaccination Resources for health Professionals. Available at: https://www.cdc.gov/flu/professionals/vaccination/index. htm. Accessed August 25, 2020.

26. Hocker S, Nagarajan E, Rubin M, et al. Clinical factors associated with Guillain-Barré syndrome following surgery. Neurol Clin Pract 2018;8(3):201–6.

27. Ropper AH, Shahani BT. Pain in Guillain-Barré syndrome. Arch Neurol 1984; 41(5):511–4.

28. Moulin DE, Hagen N, Feasby TE, et al. Pain in Guillain-Barré syndrome. Neurology 1997;48(2):328–31.

29. Pentland B, Donald SM. Pain in the Guillain-Barré syndrome: a clinical review. Pain 1994;59(2):159–64.

30. Ruts L, Drenthen J, Jongen JL, et al. Pain in Guillain-Barre syndrome: a long-term follow-up study. Neurology 2010;75(16):1439–47.

31. Willison HJ, Jacobs BC, van Doorn PA. Guillain-Barré syndrome. Lancet 2016; 388(10045):717–27.
32. van den Berg B, Fokke C, Drenthen J, et al. Paraparetic Guillain-Barré syndrome. Neurology 2014;82(22):1984–9.
33. Fokke C, van den Berg B, Drenthen J, et al. Diagnosis of Guillain-Barré syndrome and validation of Brighton criteria. Brain 2014;137(Pt 1):33–43.
34. Zochodne DW. Autonomic involvement in Guillain-Barré syndrome: a review. Muscle Nerve 1994;17(10):1145–55.
35. van Doorn PA, Ruts L, Jacobs BC. Clinical features, pathogenesis, and treatment of Guillain-Barré syndrome. Lancet Neurol 2008;7(10):939–50.
36. Islam Z, Papri N, Ara G, et al. Risk factors for respiratory failure in Guillain-Barré syndrome in Bangladesh: a prospective study. Ann Clin Transl Neurol 2019;6(2): 324–32.
37. Asbury AK, Cornblath DR. Assessment of current diagnostic criteria for Guillain-Barré syndrome. Ann Neurol 1990;27(Suppl):S21–4.
38. Walgaard C, Lingsma HF, Ruts L, et al. Prediction of respiratory insufficiency in Guillain-Barré syndrome. Ann Neurol 2010;67(6):781–7.
39. Sharshar T, Chevret S, Bourdain F, et al. Early predictors of mechanical ventilation in Guillain-Barré syndrome. Crit Care Med 2003;31(1):278–83.
40. Van der Meché FG, Van Doorn PA, Meulstee J, et al. Diagnostic and classification criteria for the Guillain-Barré syndrome. Eur Neurol 2001;45(3):133–9.
41. Albers JW, Donofrio PD, McGonagle TK. Sequential electrodiagnostic abnormalities in acute inflammatory demyelinating polyradiculoneuropathy. Muscle Nerve 1985;8(6):528–39.
42. Fisher M. An unusual variant of acute idiopathic polyneuritis (syndrome of ophthalmoplegia, ataxia and areflexia). N Engl J Med 1956;255(2):57–65.
43. Mori M, Kuwabara S, Yuki N. Fisher syndrome: clinical features, immunopathogenesis and management. Expert Rev Neurother 2012;12(1):39–51.
44. Hughes R, Léger JM. The discovery of the Guillain-Barré syndrome and related disorders. Presse Med 2013;42(6 Pt 2):e177–9.
45. Wakerley BR, Yuki N. Mimics and chameleons in Guillain-Barré and miller Fisher syndromes. Pract Neurol 2015;15(2):90–9.
46. Thornton CA, Latif AS, Emmanuel JC. Guillain-Barré syndrome associated with human immunodeficiency virus infection in Zimbabwe. Neurology 1991;41(6): 812–5.
47. Wong AH, Umapathi T, Nishimoto Y, et al. Cytoalbuminologic dissociation in asian patients with Guillain-Barré and miller Fisher syndromes. J Peripher Nerv Syst 2015;20(1):47–51.
48. Bourque PR, Brooks J, Warman-Chardon J, et al. Cerebrospinal fluid total protein in Guillain-Barré syndrome variants: correlations with clinical category, severity, and electrophysiology. J Neurol 2020;267(3):746–51.
49. Norris FH, Burns W, U KS, et al. Spinal fluid cells and protein in amyotrophic lateral sclerosis. Arch Neurol 1993;50(5):489–91.
50. Kobessho H, Oishi K, Hamaguchi H, et al. Elevation of cerebrospinal fluid protein in patients with diabetes mellitus is associated with duration of diabetes. Eur Neurol 2008;60(3):132–6.
51. Griffin JW, Li CY, Ho TW, et al. Guillain-Barré syndrome in northern China. The spectrum of neuropathological changes in clinically defined cases. Brain 1995;118(Pt 3):577–95.
52. Feasby TE, Gilbert JJ, Brown WF, et al. An acute axonal form of Guillain-Barré polyneuropathy. Brain 1986;109(Pt 6):1115–26.

53. Kalita J, Misra UK, Goyal G, et al. Guillain-Barré syndrome: subtypes and pre-
    dictors of outcome from India. J Peripher Nerv Syst 2014;19(1):36–43.
54. Hadden RD, Cornblath DR, Hughes RA, et al. Electrophysiological classification
    of Guillain-Barré syndrome: clinical associations and outcome. Plasma ex-
    change/Sandoglobulin Guillain-Barré syndrome trial Group. Ann Neurol 1998;
    44(5):780–8.
55. Ye Y, Wang K, Deng F, et al. Electrophysiological subtypes and prognosis of
    Guillain-Barré syndrome in northeastern China. Muscle Nerve 2013;47(1):68–71.
56. Wakerley BR, Uncini A, Yuki N. Guillain-Barré and Miller Fisher syndromes–new
    diagnostic classification. Nat Rev Neurol 2014;10(9):537–44.
57. DePinho RA. The age of cancer. Nature 2000;408(6809):248–54.
58. Chiba A, Kusunoki S, Shimizu T, et al. Serum IgG antibody to ganglioside GQ1b
    is a possible marker of Miller Fisher syndrome. Ann Neurol 1992;31(6):677–9.
59. Posner JB, Ertel NH, Kossmann RJ, et al. Hyponatremia in acute polyneurop-
    athy. Four cases with the syndrome of inappropriate secretion of antidiuretic hor-
    mone. Arch Neurol 1967;17(5):530–41.
60. Saifudheen K, Jose J, Gafoor VA, et al. Guillain-Barre syndrome and SIADH.
    Neurology 2011;76(8):701–4.
61. Filippatos TD, Makri A, Elisaf MS, et al. Hyponatremia in the elderly: challenges
    and solutions. Clin Interv Aging 2017;12:1957–65.
62. Haymaker WE, Kernohan JW. The Landry-Guillain-Barré syndrome; a clinico-
    pathologic report of 50 fatal cases and a critique of the literature. Medicine (Bal-
    timore) 1949;28(1):59–141.
63. Prineas JW. Pathology of the Guillain-Barré syndrome. Ann Neurol 1981;
    9(Suppl):6–19.
64. Winer JB, Hughes RA, Anderson MJ, et al. A prospective study of acute idio-
    pathic neuropathy. II. Antecedent events. J Neurol Neurosurg Psychiatry
    1988;51(5):613–8.
65. Truax BT. Autonomic disturbances in the Guillain-Barre syndrome. Semin Neurol
    1984;4(4):462–8.
66. Hughes RA. Plasma exchange versus intravenous immunoglobulin for Guillain-
    Barré syndrome. Ther Apher 1997;1(2):129–30.
67. Group TG-BsS. Plasmapheresis and acute Guillain-Barré syndrome. The Guil-
    lain-Barré syndrome study Group. Neurology 1985;35(8):1096–104.
68. Hughes RA, Swan AV, van Doorn PA. Intravenous immunoglobulin for Guillain-
    Barré syndrome. Cochrane Database Syst Rev 2014;2014(9):Cd002063.
69. van der Meché FG, Schmitz PI. A randomized trial comparing intravenous im-
    mune globulin and plasma exchange in Guillain-Barré syndrome. Dutch Guil-
    lain-Barré Study Group. N Engl J Med 1992;326(17):1123–9.
70. Cheng MJ, Christmas C. Special considerations with the use of intravenous
    immunoglobulin in older persons. Drugs Aging 2011;28(9):729–36.
71. Hughes RA, Swan AV, Raphaël JC, et al. Immunotherapy for Guillain-Barré syn-
    drome: a systematic review. Brain 2007;130(Pt 9):2245–57.
72. van Koningsveld R, Schmitz PI, Meché FG, et al. Effect of methylprednisolone
    when added to standard treatment with intravenous immunoglobulin for Guil-
    lain-Barré syndrome: randomised trial. Lancet 2004;363(9404):192–6.
73. Oczko-Walker M, Manousakis G, Wang S, et al. Plasma exchange after initial
    intravenous immunoglobulin treatment in Guillain-Barré syndrome: critical reas-
    sessment of effectiveness and cost-efficiency. J Clin Neuromuscul Dis 2010;
    12(2):55–61.

74. Lemaire A, Parquet N, Galicier L, et al. Plasma exchange in the intensive care unit: Technical aspects and complications. J Clin Apher 2017;32(6):405–12.
75. Basic-Jukic N, Brunetta B, Kes P. Plasma exchange in elderly patients. Ther Apher Dial 2010;14(2):161–5.
76. Verboon C, Doets AY, Galassi G, et al. Current treatment practice of Guillain-Barré syndrome. Neurology 2019;93(1):e59–76.
77. Simatos Arsenault N, Vincent PO, Yu BH, et al. Influence of exercise on patients with Guillain-Barré syndrome: a systematic review. Physiother Can 2016;68(4):367–76.
78. Meythaler JM, DeVivo MJ, Braswell WC. Rehabilitation outcomes of patients who have developed Guillain-Barré syndrome. Am J Phys Med Rehabil 1997;76(5):411–9.
79. Darweesh SK, Polinder S, Mulder MJ, et al. Health-related quality of life in Guillain-Barré syndrome patients: a systematic review. J Peripher Nerv Syst 2014;19(1):24–35.
80. Liu J, Wang LN, McNicol ED. Pharmacological treatment for pain in Guillain-Barré syndrome. Cochrane Database Syst Rev 2015;2015(4):Cd009950.
81. de Vries JM, Hagemans ML, Bussmann JB, et al. Fatigue in neuromuscular disorders: focus on Guillain-Barré syndrome and Pompe disease. Cell Mol Life Sci 2010;67(5):701–13.
82. Das A, Kalita J, Misra UK. Recurrent Guillain Barre' syndrome. Electromyogr Clin Neurophysiol 2004;44(2):95–102.
83. Kuitwaard K, van Koningsveld R, Ruts L, et al. Recurrent Guillain-Barré syndrome. J Neurol Neurosurg Psychiatry 2009;80(1):56–9.
84. Mossberg N, Nordin M, Movitz C, et al. The recurrent Guillain-Barré syndrome: a long-term population-based study. Acta Neurol Scand 2012;126(3):154–61.
85. Sung JY, Tani J, Park SB, et al. Early identification of 'acute-onset' chronic inflammatory demyelinating polyneuropathy. Brain 2014;137(Pt 8):2155–63.
86. McCombe PA, Pollard JD, McLeod JG. Chronic inflammatory demyelinating polyradiculoneuropathy. A clinical and electrophysiological study of 92 cases. Brain 1987;110(Pt 6):1617–30.
87. Mathey EK, Park SB, Hughes RA, et al. Chronic inflammatory demyelinating polyradiculoneuropathy: from pathology to phenotype. J Neurol Neurosurg Psychiatry 2015;86(9):973–85.
88. Kleyweg RP, van der Meché FG. Treatment related fluctuations in Guillain-Barré syndrome after high-dose immunoglobulins or plasma-exchange. J Neurol Neurosurg Psychiatry 1991;54(11):957–60.
89. Ropper AE, Albert JW, Addison R. Limited relapse in Guillain-Barré syndrome after plasma exchange. Arch Neurol 1988;45(3):314–5.
90. Ruts L, Drenthen J, Jacobs BC, et al. Distinguishing acute-onset CIDP from fluctuating Guillain-Barre syndrome: a prospective study. Neurology 2010;74(21):1680–6.
91. Ruts L, van Koningsveld R, van Doorn PA. Distinguishing acute-onset CIDP from Guillain-Barré syndrome with treatment related fluctuations. Neurology 2005;65(1):138–40.
92. van den Berg B, Storm EF, Garssen MJP, et al. Clinical outcome of Guillain-Barré syndrome after prolonged mechanical ventilation. J Neurol Neurosurg Psychiatry 2018;89(9):949–54.
93. van den Berg B, Bunschoten C, van Doorn PA, et al. Mortality in Guillain-Barre syndrome. Neurology 2013;80(18):1650–4.

94. Wong AH, Umapathi T, Shahrizaila N, et al. The value of comparing mortality of Guillain-Barré syndrome across different regions. J Neurol Sci 2014; 344(1–2):60–2.

95. Forsberg A, Press R, Holmqvist LW. Residual disability 10 years after falling ill in Guillain-Barré syndrome: a prospective follow-up study. J Neurol Sci 2012; 317(1–2):74–9.

96. Dornonville de la Cour C, Jakobsen J. Residual neuropathy in long-term population-based follow-up of Guillain-Barré syndrome. Neurology 2005;64(2): 246–53.

97. Garssen MP, Van Koningsveld R, Van Doorn PA. Residual fatigue is independent of antecedent events and disease severity in Guillain-Barré syndrome. J Neurol 2006;253(9):1143–6.

98. Rekand T, Gramstad A, Vedeler CA. Fatigue, pain and muscle weakness are frequent after Guillain-Barré syndrome and poliomyelitis. J Neurol 2009; 256(3):349–54.

99. Garssen MP, Bussmann JB, Schmitz PI, et al. Physical training and fatigue, fitness, and quality of life in Guillain-Barré syndrome and CIDP. Neurology 2004;63(12):2393–5.

100. Moalem-Taylor G, Allbutt HN, Iordanova MD, et al. Pain hypersensitivity in rats with experimental autoimmune neuritis, an animal model of human inflammatory demyelinating neuropathy. Brain Behav Immun 2007;21(5):699–710.

101. Hughes RA, Wijdicks EF, Benson E, et al. Supportive care for patients with Guillain-Barré syndrome. Arch Neurol 2005;62(8):1194–8.

102. Bernsen RA, de Jager AE, Kuijer W, et al. Psychosocial dysfunction in the first year after Guillain-Barré syndrome. Muscle Nerve 2010;41(4):533–9.

Chronic Immune-Mediated Polyneuropathies

Stephen Zachary Cox, DO, Kelly G. Gwathmey, MD*

KEYWORDS

- CIDP • Multifocal motor neuropathy
- Multifocal acquired sensory and motor polyneuropathy • Vasculitic neuropathy

KEY POINTS

- Chronic inflammatory demyelinating polyradiculoneuropathy (CIDP) typically presents with progressive generalized weakness and large fiber sensory deficit.
- CIDP is a treatable neuropathy and responds to intravenous immune globulins, subcutaneous immune globulins, corticosteroids, and plasma exchange in most cases.
- Vasculitic neuropathies present with painful, progressive, sensory, and motor mononeuropathies.
- Failure to identify and treat chronic immune-mediated polyneuropathies may result in significant disability and even death.

INTRODUCTION

Immune-mediated chronic polyneuropathies include a diverse group of diseases that can vary widely in clinical presentation and pathophysiology. For those patients affected, these diseases represent a significant source of disability, often requiring life-long therapy to prevent significant complications. This article focuses first on chronic inflammatory demyelinating polyradiculoneuropathy (CIDP) and its variants, followed by vasculitic neuropathies, both systemic and nonsystemic with attention to clinical presentation, initial workup, pathophysiology, and treatment options. This discussion does not include other microvasculitic processes such as diabetic and nondiabetic lumbosacral radiculoplexus neuropathies. Other chronic inflammatory neuropathies associated with rheumatological disorders and systemic inflammatory diseases are briefly highlighted in **Table 1**.

Department of Neurology, Virginia Commonwealth University, 1101 East Marshall Street, PO Box 980599, Richmond, VA 23298, USA
* Corresponding author.
E-mail address: Kelly.gwathmey@vcuhealth.org

Clin Geriatr Med 37 (2021) 327–345
https://doi.org/10.1016/j.cger.2021.01.006
0749-0690/21/© 2021 Elsevier Inc. All rights reserved.

geriatric.theclinics.com

Table 1
Other causes of chronic immune-mediated polyneuropathies

Connective Tissue Diseases

• Sjögren Syndrome	• SFN • Sensory ataxic neuropathy (ie, sensory neuronopathy or dorsal root ganglionopathy) • Sensorimotor axonal polyneuropathy • Demyelinating polyneuropathy • Vasculitic neuropathy • Polyradiculoneuropathy • Autonomic neuropathy	• ANA • Anti-SSA, anti-SSB antibodies • Anticentromere antibodies • Schirmer test, Rose Bengal testing (ocular surface staining), salivary flow study, labial salivary gland biopsy if indicated	• Consider IVIg for SFN,[60,61] sensory ataxic neuropathy,[62] demyelinating neuropathy, sensorimotor neuropathy, and autonomic neuropathy[63] • Corticosteroid benefit unclear although may be helpful in large fiber neuropathies, sensory ataxic neuropathies (with IVIg)[62] • Rituximab often considered if IVIg refractory[63–65] • Other treatments used: mycophenolate mofetil, azathioprine, cyclophosphamide, tacrolimus, plasma exchange
• Systemic Lupus Erythematosus	• Large fiber sensory polyneuropathy • SFN • Vasculitic neuropathy	• ANA • Anti–double stranded DNA • Anti-Smith antibodies • Antiphospholipid antibodies • C3 and C4 or CH50 complement levels • ESR • CRP • Urine protein-to-creatinine ratio	• Corticosteroids for large fiber neuropathy[66,67] • Other agents used: azathioprine, cyclophosphamide, mycophenolate mofetil • Treatment of SFN unknown
• Rheumatoid Arthritis	• Large fiber sensory or sensorimotor polyneuropathy • Mononeuropathy (eg, carpal tunnel syndrome) • Vasculitic neuropathy	• Joint involvement as per 2010 ACR/EULAR criteria[68] • Rheumatoid factor • Anticitrullinated peptide/protein antibody • ESR • CRP	• Unknown treatment of large fiber polyneuropathy • Splinting, corticosteroid injection, surgical decompression for median mononeuropathy at the wrist (carpal tunnel syndrome) • Glucocorticoids and cyclophosphamide

(continued on next page)

Table 1
(continued)

			for vasculitic neuropathy[69,70]
• Scleroderma (Systemic Sclerosis)	• Large fiber sensory or sensorimotor polyneuropathy • Mononeuropathy	• ANA • Anti-DNA topoisomerase I (Scl-70) • Anticentromere antibody • Anti-RNA polymerase III antibody	• Unknown treatment of large fiber polyneuropathy • Splinting, corticosteroid injection, surgical decompression for median mononeuropathy
Sarcoidosis	• SFN • Large fiber sensory and sensorimotor polyneuropathy • Polyradiculoneuropathy • Mononeuropathy • Vasculitic neuropathy	• Angiotensin-converting enzyme • Soluble interleukin-2 receptor level • Chest radiograph • Pulmonary function testing • Ophthalmic evaluation with slit lamp • Skin examination and referral to dermatology as needed • Occasionally FDG-PET, Gallium 67 scanning • Tissue biopsy demonstrating noncaseating granulomas	• For SFN, response to standard immunomodulating therapies such as methotrexate and corticosteroids is often poor[71] • IVIg and infliximab may be helpful • For large fiber and multiple mononeuropathies likely corticosteroids are helpful[72–74]
Behcet Disease	• Large fiber sensory or sensorimotor polyneuropathy • Vasculitic neuropathy	• Diagnosis relies on presences of recurrent oral and genital ulcers, anterior or posterior uveitis, retinal vasculitis, skin lesions (pseudofolliculitis, erythema nodosum, papulopustular lesions, acneiform nodules) and positive pathergy test	• Unclear, given the rarity of peripheral nervous system manifestations. • Extrapolating from therapies used in parenchymal involvement, corticosteroids, interferon-α, azathioprine, methotrexate, TNF-α antagonists, and cyclophosphamide could be considered.[75]

Immune-mediated Gastrointestinal Disorders

• Inflammatory Bowel Disease (Crohn Disease and Ulcerative Colitis)	• Demyelinating polyneuropathy • SFN • Large fiber sensorimotor polyneuropathy	• Small bowel imaging with MRI (Crohn disease) • Endoscopy with mucosal biopsies	• Corticosteroids[76] • IVIg • Plasma exchange

(continued on next page)

Table 1 (continued)			
	• Radiculoplexus neuropathy		
• Celiac Disease	• SFN • Large fiber sensorimotor polyneuropathy	• Antigliadin, antitissue transglutaminase, antiendomysial antibodies • Villous atrophy on small bowel biopsy	• Gluten avoidance[76] • Exclude other causes (vitamin deficiencies) • Mixed results with immunomodulatory therapy

Abbreviations: ANA, antinuclear antibody; anti-SSA, anti-Sjogren syndrome antibody A; anti-SSB, anti-Sjogren syndrome antibody B; CRP, C-reactive protein; ESR, erythrocyte sedimentation rate; FDG-PET, fluorodeoxyglucose positron emission tomography; IVIg, intravenous immune globulins; SFN, small fiber neuropathy.

*Although not explicitly stated in Table 1, basic laboratory studies (see **Box 1**) and electrodiagnostic studies should be performed in all patients. Should electrodiagnostic studies be normal, then a skin biopsy looking for reduced intraepidermal nerve fiber density supporting a small fiber neuropathy should be performed. On occasion, autonomic testing is pursued in those with significant dysautonomia or to support a diagnosis of small fiber neuropathy.

CHRONIC INFLAMMATORY DEMYELINATING POLYRADICULONEUROPATHY
History/Background

CIDP was first described in 1890 by Eichhorst as episodes of "recurrent neuritis" although the term chronic immune demyelinating polyradiculoneuropathy would not be coined until almost a century later.[1] Current estimates of the incidence rate of CIDP is at 0.33 per 100,000 and the prevalence rate at 2.81 per 100,000.[2] Despite its relative rarity it is the most common chronic autoimmune neuropathy. The age of onset of CIDP is variable occurring from childhood to late in adulthood. Even when symptoms do begin at an early age, many patients experience a relapsing/remitting or progressive course that requires lifelong therapy and results in significant disability.

Pathophysiology

CIDP is the result of the immune-mediated destruction of peripheral nerve myelin. The exact mechanisms by which this occurs are not yet fully understood but likely comprise a mixture of cellular and humoral immunity.[3] T-cell and macrophage infiltration is seen on biopsy with phagocytosis of peripheral nerve myelin.[4,5] Consequently, heavily myelinated peripheral nerves are the most affected in this condition.

Presentation and Examination Findings

CIDP is characterized by insidious onset, symmetric, generalized weakness, and large fiber sensory dysfunction. Patients often develop a sensory ataxia due to the involvement of proprioceptive fibers. Other symptoms include neuropathic pain, postural tremor as well as significant fatigue although weakness should be the predominate feature of the disease.[6,7] Examination reveals symmetric weakness, both proximal and distal, diminished vibratory and proprioceptive sensation, and perhaps most importantly the depression or altogether absence of deep tendon reflexes. Patients may have a monophasic, relapsing/remitting, or chronically progressive course.

Several characteristics help distinguish CIDP from Guillain-Barré syndrome (GBS), a condition similar in pathogenesis and presentation. Unlike GBS, a prodromal illness is

---

Box 1
Recommended laboratory studies for those with suspected immune-mediated polyneuropathies

Initial Serum Laboratory Studies
  Complete blood count with differential
  Basic metabolic panel
  Liver function tests
  Hemoglobin A1c or glucose tolerance test
  Thyroid function tests
  B12, methylmalonic acid
  Serum and urine electrophoresis
  Immunofixation
  Serum light chains
  ESR and CRP
  Hepatitis serologies
  Antinuclear antibodies
  Antineutrophil cytoplasmic antibodies
  Rheumatoid factor

Abbreviations: CRP, C-reactive protein; ESR, erythrocyte sedimentation rate.

---

not a defining feature of CIDP. The timing surrounding onset and nadir of symptoms is a key factor in differentiating CIDP from GBS. Patients with CIDP reach the nadir of their sensory and motor symptoms at or after 8 weeks following symptom onset. The initiation of symptoms tends to be more gradual as well, although a subset of patients will have an abrupt onset and are termed acute-onset CIDP or A-CIDP.[8] Cranial nerve, bulbar involvement, and autonomic disturbance are more common in GBS as opposed to CIDP.

Evaluation

Although the clinical presentation and examination should strongly support the diagnosis of CIDP, further investigation may be warranted, including serum, cerebrospinal fluid (CSF), electrodiagnostic, imaging, and rarely histopathology. Initial serum laboratories should be performed to exclude alternative causes. For a list of appropriate initial laboratory testing in all suspected immune-mediated polyneuropathies please refer to **Box 1**. The presence of a monoclonal gammopathy or other paraprotein disorder may prompt further testing, which is discussed in Leavell and Shin's article, "Paraproteinemias and Peripheral Nerve Disease," in this issue.

    CSF studies can often be deferred in straightforward cases of CIDP. If obtained, the most common finding is albuminocytological dissociation (elevated protein in setting of a normal leukocyte count). The sensitivity of this finding is traditionally quite high at 95%, although there is recent evidence to suggest that increasing the protein upper limit of normal value may improve specificity at a modest cost to sensitivity[9]. Alternative diagnoses should be considered if CSF studies reveal a pleocytosis.

    Electrodiagnostic studies including nerve conduction studies and electromyography are mandatory to confirm a diagnosis of CIDP. Electrodiagnostic studies show evidence of slowed conduction velocities, conduction block, temporal dispersion, prolonged distal latencies, as well as prolonged or absent F waves and H reflexes. All of these findings are consistent with a peripheral demyelinating process. CIDP variants may have unique electrodiagnostic features. **Table 2** reviews the clinical presentation, diagnosis, and treatment of the CIDP variants.

Table 2
Chronic inflammatory demyelinating polyradiculoneuropathy variants

	Clinical Features	Electrodiagnostic Studies	Treatment	Other
Sensory CIDP	Symmetric sensory loss without clinical weakness, early upper extremity involvement, cranial nerve involvement[77]	• Studies typically show evidence of motor nerve involvement[78]	• Corticosteroids • IVIg • Plasma exchange	• May go on to develop weakness and typical CIDP
Motor CIDP	Symmetric weakness with absence of sensory symptoms	• Can completely spare sensory nerves or may have mild evidence of sensory nerve involvement	• Poor response to steroids[79] • Can use IVIg or plasma exchange	• May represent a spectrum including multifocal motor neuropathy
Distal Acquired Demyelinating Sensory Neuropathy (DADS)	Distal sensory loss resulting in ataxia and mild distal motor involvement May have action tremor	• Disproportionate slowing of distal motor conduction velocity, no conduction block, and absent sural responses[80]	• Poor response to IVIg, plasma exchange, and corticosteroids in the presence of MAG antibodies • Possibly responsive to rituximab[19]	• Often associated with IgM monoclonal gammopathy and MAG antibodies
Multifocal Acquired Demyelinating Sensory and Motor Neuropathy (MADSAM)	Multifocal, asymmetrical motor and sensory involvement, which may include cranial neuropathies[20]	• Similar to typical CIDP	• Corticosteroids • IVIg • Plasma exchange	• Almost 50% will progress to typical CIDP • Also known as Lewis-Sumner syndrome
Chronic Immune Sensory Polyneuropathy (CISP)	Similar presentation to sensory CIDP with prominent sensory ataxia	• Normal nerve conduction studies[81] • Somatosensory evoked potentials will be abnormal	• Corticosteroids • IVIg	• MRI may demonstrate enlarged, contrast-enhancing nerve roots • CSF analysis may demonstrate elevated protein • Considered a subclassification of sensory CIDP

Abbreviations: CISP, chronic immune sensory polyneuropathy; DADS, distal acquired demyelinating sensory neuropathy; IVIg, intravenous immune globulins;

Imaging is not routinely performed in the evaluation of CIDP although certain abnormalities may support the diagnosis. Enlargement of peripheral nerves, nerve roots, and plexuses with contrast enhancement may be seen on MRI.[10] Focal enlargement of peripheral nerves, particularly in the early stages of disease, may appear on ultrasound.

Nerve biopsy is very rarely undertaken if the suspected diagnosis is CIDP, as the clinical presentation and electrodiagnostic testing are usually sufficient to make the diagnosis. However, in atypical presentations that do not clearly fit into established categories, biopsy may be required. The hallmark histopathologic findings on nerve biopsy are evidence of chronic demyelination and remyelination resulting in an onion bulb appearance along with epineurial, endoneurial, or perivascular macrophage and T cell infiltration (**Fig. 1**).[4]

Treatment

First-line therapy for CIDP includes intravenous or subcutaneous immunoglobulin (IVIg and SCIg, respectively), plasma exchange, and corticosteroids. Treatment is generally conducted in a 2-fold approach with an induction phase followed by maintenance therapy. Response varies individually particularly between CIDP variants as discussed in **Table 2**. Overall response rate is 50% to 70%.[11] Medical comorbidities, severity of disease, patient preferences, and response to treatment help guide therapeutic choices. Response can be measured in a variety of ways. Muscle strength, particularly grip strength, as measured on examination is a useful metric commonly used. There exist standardized scales such as the Inflammatory Neuropathy Cause and Treatment disability score as well as the more recent Inflammatory Rasch-built Overall Disability Scale. These measures, coupled with patient-reported quality of life measures, help build a more comprehensive picture for providers to judge success of therapies.

IVIg is a mainstay of CIDP treatment both for induction and maintenance therapy and received Food and Drug Administration (FDA) approval for this indication in 2008. Induction therapy is dosed at 2 g/kg divided over 2 to 5 days. There is currently no clear evidence for optimal maintenance dosing but typically a dose of 1 g/kg every 3 weeks is used after initial induction.[12] A full 6 weeks should be given to assess response to therapy before alternative therapies are considered.[13] Dosing considerations for continued maintenance should be made with treatment response in mind and weaning the frequency of administration as well as the dose received with each infusion is reasonable provided symptoms remain stable. A recent alternative to IVIg was approved by the FDA in 2018 in the form of SCIg, which offers patients the option of self-administering the subcutaneous form on a weekly basis rather than having to go to an infusion center. SCIg has been found to be comparable to IV formulation in prevention of relapses although onset of improvement may lag in treatment-naïve patients.[14,15] Side effects of Ig therapy include headache, nausea, fatigue, and increased risk of thrombotic events. Many of these side effects can be mitigated simply by slowing the infusion rate or decreasing the concentration of the agent being used. If necessary, premedication based on the type and severity of the reaction can be considered and may include acetaminophen, diphenhydramine, or IV corticosteroids.

Plasma exchange has shown equal efficacy when compared with IVIg, and therapy is carried out in a similar fashion with induction phase followed by maintenance dosing.[16] Induction is carried out in 5 to 10 exchanges of 50 mL/kg alternating days during the first 2 to 4 weeks, followed by 1 to 2 exchanges monthly or even as frequent as every 3 weeks. Because there is no active medication being administered, it is generally well tolerated. However, as dialysis, patients can have complications based around the large amount of fluid shifts with treatments. Permanent central venous

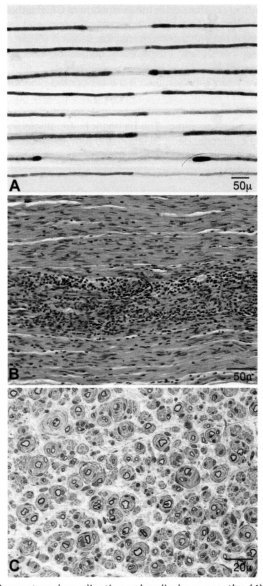

Fig. 1. Chronic inflammatory demyelinating polyradiculoneuropathy. (*A*) Teased fiber preparations from a sural nerve showing multiple segments of segmental demyelination. (*B*) Longitudinal paraffin section (stained with hematoxylin and eosin) from a sciatic biopsy showing large endoneurial perivascular mononuclear cell infiltration. (*C*) Epoxy cross-section (stained with methylene blue) from the sural nerve showing widespread hypertrophic neuropathy with onion-bulb formation (stacks of Schwann cell cytoplasmic processes) and thin myelin. (Reused with permission from Mayo Clin Proc. 2018 Jun;93(6):777-793.)

access is required and can present its own set of challenges and complications. These issues, coupled with the frequency of maintenance therapy, tend to relegate plasma exchange to those patients who have failed or could not tolerate therapy with Ig.

Corticosteroids are used as induction therapy and, if possible, avoided for maintenance given the significant adverse effects associated with chronic use. Multiple options both in dosing and agent can be considered. Oral prednisone at a dose of 1 to 1.5 mg/kg every 24 to 48 hours, IV methylprednisolone weekly, or oral dexamethasone, 40 mg, for 4 days repeated every 4 weeks can all be considered and have been shown to have equal efficacy and safety.[17] Patients with refractory disease or who cannot tolerate other therapies may require long-term steroid treatment. Steroid-sparing agents are often considered in these cases; unfortunately, data backing the efficacy of many of these medications are lacking.[18]

If a patient is refractory to these 3 therapeutic options, reevaluation is warranted to exclude another diagnosis provided they have received an adequate trial. As mentioned earlier IVIg should be allowed 6 weeks to assess response. Plasma exchange and corticosteroids tend to have more rapid onset although again induction for plasma exchange may take place over 4 weeks. The decision to switch therapy should also be weighed with the clinical picture of the patient in mind. More aggressive disease may require more frequent reconsideration of therapeutic options.

Chronic Inflammatory Demyelinating Polyradiculoneuropathy Variants

Distal acquired demyelinating symmetric neuropathy (DADS) is a CIDP variant characterized by, as the name implies, a distally predominant, symmetric sensory and motor neuropathy. Sensory symptoms tend to predominant often resulting in an ataxia, and when motor symptoms are present, they are typically mild and involve the distal lower extremities. DADS is associated with anti–myelin-associated glycoprotein antibodies and a high rate of IgM monoclonal gammopathy (reference paraprotein disorders and peripheral nerve disease). This may correspond to its relative refractory nature to traditional first-line agents. Rituximab may offer benefit.[19]

Multifocal acquired demyelinating sensory and motor neuropathy, otherwise known as Lewis-Sumner syndrome, is another CIDP variant distinct in its asymmetric presentation. Similar to traditional CIDP, both motor and sensory nerve involvement is present although symptoms predominate in upper extremities.[20] Cranial nerve involvement can also be seen. Nearly half of the patients will progress to CIDP.

There are many other variants of CIDP, including those with varying degrees of sensory or motor symptoms. Treatment approach is overall similar to traditional CIDP with some notable exceptions. Although treatment is the same, response to therapy can differ between variants. Please refer to **Table 2** for a list of variants along with associated presentations, electrophysiologic findings, and treatment options.

Multifocal Motor Neuropathy and Nodo-Paranodopathies

Nodo-paranodopathies may present similarly to CIDP, but underlying pathophysiology is not a demyelinating process but rather the production of antibodies to targets on or near the Nodes of Ranvier.[21] One such entity is multifocal motor neuropathy (MMN), a disorder that until recently was characterized as a CIDP variant until its pathophysiology was more clearly understood.[22] MMN is a result of autoantibodies to ganglioside GM1, which tends to be concentrated at peripheral motor nerve nodes.[23] It is characterized by the presence of multiple motor mononeuropathies in an asymmetric, distal-predominant pattern with the presence of fasciculations and cramping. First-line treatment is IVIG, and MMN is known for its poor response to plasma exchange and corticosteroids.[12] There exist now multiple other identified antigens that serve as autoimmune targets at or adjacent to peripheral nerve nodes. These include contactin-1, contactin-associated protein-1, and neurofascin-155.[24] As with MMN, treatment response differs from traditional CIDP, and other therapeutic options such as rituximab or cyclophosphamide may be considered.[25,26]

VASCULITIC NEUROPATHIES
Background/Definitions

Regardless of the underlying cause, vasculitic neuropathies result from inflammatory infiltration of the vasa nervorum, the blood vessels that supply the peripheral nerves. The resulting ischemic injury of the peripheral nerves results in pain, weakness, and numbness. Several vasculitic neuropathy classification systems exist, which catalog these disorders in terms of size of the affected vessels and underlying cause.[27] These neuropathies may be associated with primary systemic vasculitis, in which vasculitis affects multiple organs without alternative autoimmune cause (eg, eosinophilic granulomatosis with polyangiitis). Vasculitic neuropathies may also be secondary to underlying rheumatological conditions, malignancy, infections, or rarely drug exposure. When the inflammation is restricted to the peripheral nerves it is considered nonsystemic vasculitic neuropathy (NSVN). Please see **Table 3** for a list of the underlying causes of vasculitic neuropathies.

Presentation and Examination Findings

The archetypal presentation with vasculitic neuropathies is that of mononeuritis multiplex characterized by acute to subacute painful sensorimotor mononeuropathies (eg, painful wrist drop due to radial mononeuropathy, followed by painful foot drop from common fibular mononeuropathy). These mononeuropathies occur in a nonlength-dependent, asymmetrical pattern, although often eventually overlap, conforming to a distal symmetric or asymmetrical polyneuropathy pattern. Taking a careful history and obtaining an account of multiple painful mononeuropathies is imperative. Those with systemic vasculitic neuropathy typically have a stepwise progression, whereas those with NSVN may progress more slowly, resulting in diagnostic delay. In those with systemic vasculitis, involvement of other organs, such as the lungs, skin, kidneys, and gastrointestinal tract, is expected. In addition, constitutional symptoms are commonplace, including weight loss, fatigue, arthralgias, and myalgias. These symptoms, however, are rarely encountered when the vasculitis is isolated to the peripheral nerves.

Evaluation

In any patient with suspected vasculitic neuropathy, a comprehensive panel of laboratory studies must be completed (see **Box 1**). If the patient has an erythrocyte sedimentation rate (ESR) greater than 100 mm/h and antineutrophil cytoplasmic antibody (ANCA) positivity, this highly suggests primary systemic vasculitic neuropathy.[28] Mildly elevated ESR may also be encountered in NSVN in approximately 70% of cases.[29]

Electrodiagnostic testing serves several important roles in the evaluation of those with suspected vasculitic neuropathy. Identification of a multiple mononeuropathies or asymmetrical axonal sensorimotor polyneuropathy is highly consistent with vasculitic neuropathy in the appropriate clinical setting.[30] Also, electrodiagnostic studies may guide nerve and muscle biopsy.

A clinical suspicion of vasculitic neuropathy is one of the few indications for cutaneous nerve biopsy, and it is often mandatory in this context. Any affected cutaneous sensory nerve can be biopsied, although the sural, superficial radial, and superficial fibular are the most common. It is generally recommended to concurrently biopsy a

Table 3
Common vasculitic neuropathies

Cause of Vasculitic Neuropathy	Comments
Primary Systemic Vasculitides	
Predominantly Small Vessel Vasculitis	
Microscopic polyangiitis	• Organs involved include lungs, kidneys, skin, and abdominal pain • Commonly associated with ANCAs (MPO > PR3) • Neuropathy prevalence 40%–50%[34]
Granulomatosis with polyangiitis	• Granulomatous infiltration of the upper and lower respiratory tracts • May have kidney involvement • Commonly associated with ANCAs (PR3> MPO) • Neuropathy prevalence 15%–25%[82]
Eosinophilic granulomatosis with polyangiitis	• Associated with asthma, blood eosinophilia, paranasal sinus abnormalities, extranasal eosinophil infiltration, fleeting pulmonary infiltrates • Commonly associated with ANCAs (MPO > PR3) • Neuropathy prevalence 60%–70%[83–85]
Predominantly Medium Vessel Vasculitis	
Polyarteritis nodosa	• Frequently triggered by hepatitis B • Often skin involvement, renal involvement (renal artery aneurysms, hypertension), abdominal pain • Prevalence of neuropathy 75%[86]
Secondary Systemic Vasculitides	
Connective Tissue Disease	
Rheumatoid arthritis	• Late manifestation of severe seropositive rheumatoid arthritis • Neuropathy present in 40%–50% of rheumatoid vasculitis[69,87]
Systemic lupus erythematosus	
Sjögren syndrome	• Associated with sicca symptoms • Associated with positive anti-SSA or anti-SSB antibodies, positive antinuclear antibody • Evidence of lymphocytic infiltrates on salivary gland biopsy • Vasculitis is only one of many peripheral nerve manifestations in Sjögren
Infection	
Hepatitis C and cryoglobulinemia	• Associated symptoms include purpura, glomerulonephritis, ulceration, arthritis, and sicca symptoms[54] • Incidence of neuropathy is 65%[58,88–92]
Hepatitis B and polyarteritis nodosa	• Relatively rare with advent of hepatitis B vaccine
HIV	• Rare cause of vasculitic neuropathy
Drugs	• Associated with tumor necrosis factor inhibitors, minocycline, checkpoint inhibitors, and cocaine[93]
Malignancy	• Relatively rare • Associated with anti-Hu antibodies • Associated with lymphoma and small cell lung cancer

(continued on next page)

Table 3 (continued)	
Cause of Vasculitic Neuropathy	Comments
Nonsystemic vasculitic neuropathy	• Likely the most common form of vasculitic neuropathy • May be more gradually progressive • Not fatal

Abbreviations: ANCA, antineutrophil cytoplasmic antibody; HIV, human immunodeficiency virus; MPO, myeloperoxidase; PR3, proteinase 3; SSA, Sjögren syndrome–associated A; SSB, Sjögren syndrome–associated B.

piece of muscle, as it increases diagnostic yield to 60% to 70%.[31,32] Nerve biopsy is vital to secure the diagnosis in NSVN, whereas it can be avoided in primary systemic vasculitides if diagnostic biopsy of another organ has already occurred.

Some experts classify vasculitic neuropathies by the size of the involved vessels into either nerve large arteriole vasculitis or microvasculitis.[33] Nerve large arteriole vasculitis is present in most primary systemic and secondary systemic vasculitic neuropathies, whereas microvasculitis is often associated with NSVN and occasionally Sjögren syndrome–associated vasculitic neuropathy. Nerve large arteriole vasculitis affects vessels ranging from 75 to 300 μm and is characterized by fibrinoid necrosis of the tunica media and intima (**Fig. 2**).[34] In contrast, microvasculitis targets smaller vessels, typically less than 40 μm in diameter, including the small arterioles, capillaries, and venules. Other common histopathological features, regardless of the underlying cause, include Wallerian degeneration, perineurial thickening, neovascularization, hemosiderin-laden macrophages, and deposits of complement, fibrinogen, and IgM in the vessel walls.[28,35–40]

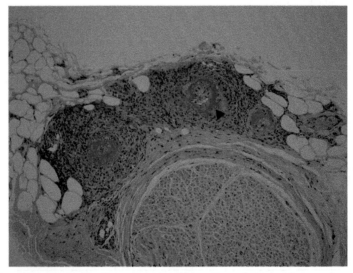

Fig. 2. Vasculitic neuropathy. Transverse paraffin section of the sural nerve demonstrating large arteriole vasculitis (hematoxylin and eosin stain). Fibrinoid necrosis is appreciated in all 3 vessels (*arrowhead*) as well as transmural inflammatory infiltration.

Treatment

The treatment approach to vasculitic neuropathy is dictated by the underlying cause. As systemic vasculitis can be deadly, aggressive treatment should be initiated promptly. Induction therapy with corticosteroids (1 mg/kg day of prednisone, occasionally preceded by several days of 1 g of IV methylprednisolone) is used for 6 to 8 weeks before a tapering.[41,42] To supplement corticosteroids, cyclophosphamide or rituximab (especially with ANCA-associated vasculitis [AAV]) may be used.[43–45] In those with AAV and milder symptoms, methotrexate may be used with corticosteroids.[46,47] Following induction therapy, maintenance therapy is achieved with oral, steroid sparing immunosuppressants such as azathioprine or methotrexate for 18 to 24 months.[48]

NSVN, although not fatal, still carries risk of permanent neurologic deficits. Experts now recommend combination therapy (corticosteroids with either cyclophosphamide or methotrexate). Rituximab may be used as the first-line alternative therapy for severe NSVN.[49]

The virus-associated vasculitic neuropathies (hepatitis C–associated cryoglobulinemia, hepatitis B–associated polyarteritis nodosa, and human immunodeficiency virus) have historically been managed with antiviral therapy. There is emerging evidence, however, that concomitant immunosuppressant or immunomodulatory therapies such as plasma exchange, rituximab, and corticosteroids may be indicated in advanced disease.[50–59]

Although addressing the neuropathic pain in vasculitic neuropathies does not alter disease trajectory, it is a cornerstone of comprehensive management. Please see Pedowitz and colleagues' article, "Management of Neuropathic Pain in the Geriatric Population," in this issue for details.

SUMMARY

The chronic immune-mediated polyneuropathies are a wide spectrum of autoimmune conditions ranging from those solely affecting the peripheral nervous system (ie, CIDP and NSVN) to those associated with systemic inflammatory conditions (eg, ANCA-associated vasculitis, sarcoidosis, or Sjögren syndrome). Much is still being discovered about these conditions and, as a result, classifications remain somewhat fluid. These polyneuropathies are characterized by their varied, unique clinical presentations. A familiarity with these disorders enables the provider to initiate the appropriate diagnostic evaluation and treatment, whereas failure to identify these conditions may result in permanent disability and even death.

CLINICS CARE POINTS

- CIDP is a demyelinating polyneuropathy characterized by symmetric, generalized sensory and motor dysfunction with areflexia on examination often with relapsing, remitting, or progressive course.

- Diagnosis is made from careful history, neurologic examination, electrodiagnostic studies, and rarely nerve biopsy.

- First-line treatment of CIDP includes corticosteroids, IVIg, and plasma exchange.

- There are many CIDP variants and closely associated conditions such as nodo-paranodopathies. Making the correct diagnosis is important for selection of appropriate therapies.

- Vasculitic neuropathies present with painful, progressive sensory and motor mononeuropathies or "mononeuritis multiplex."

- The vasculitic neuropathies may be associated with systemic vasculitis, be secondary to rheumatological conditions, infections, malignancy, or drug exposure, or isolated to the peripheral nervous system (NSVN).
- Diagnosis of vasculitic neuropathies requires taking a thorough history, the neurologic examination, extensive serum studies, electrodiagnostic studies, and often nerve biopsy.
- Treatment of the vasculitic neuropathies is primarily corticosteroids. Often cyclophosphamide, rituximab, and occasionally methotrexate are also used for induction therapy. Maintenance therapy consists of transitioning the patients to oral steroid-sparing agents.

DISCLOSURE

Dr S. Cox has nothing to disclose. Dr K.G. Gwathmey has received speaking and consulting honoraria from Alexion pharmaceuticals.

REFERENCES

1. Fadia M, Shroff S, Simpson E. Immune-mediated neuropathies. Curr Treat Options Neurol 2019;21(6):28.
2. Broers MC, Bunschoten C, Nieboer D, et al. Incidence and prevalence of chronic inflammatory demyelinating polyradiculoneuropathy: a systematic review and meta-analysis. Neuroepidemiology 2019;52(3–4):161–72.
3. Franssen H, Straver DCG. Pathophysiology of immune-mediated demyelinating neuropathies–Part II: Neurology. Muscle Nerve 2014;49(1):4–20.
4. Dyck PJ, Lais AC, Ohta M, et al. Chronic inflammatory polyradiculoneuropathy. Mayo Clin Proc 1975;50(11):621–37. Available at: http://www.ncbi.nlm.nih.gov/pubmed/1186294.
5. Kiefer R, Kieseier BC, Stoll G, et al. The role of macrophages in immune-mediated damage to the peripheral nervous system. Prog Neurobiol 2001;64(2):109–27. Available at: http://www.ncbi.nlm.nih.gov/pubmed/11240209.
6. Cao Y, Menon P, Ching-Fen Chang F, et al. Postural tremor and chronic inflammatory demyelinating polyneuropathy. Muscle Nerve 2017;55(3):338–43.
7. Merkies IS, Schmitz PI, Samijn JP, et al. Fatigue in immune-mediated polyneuropathies. European inflammatory neuropathy cause and treatment (INCAT) group. Neurology 1999;53(8):1648–54.
8. McCombe PA, Pollard JD, McLeod JG. Chronic inflammatory demyelinating polyradiculoneuropathy. A clinical and electrophysiological study of 92 cases. Brain 1987;110(Pt 6):1617–30.
9. Breiner A, Bourque PR, Allen JA. Updated cerebrospinal fluid total protein reference values improve chronic inflammatory demyelinating polyneuropathy diagnosis. Muscle Nerve 2019;60(2):180–3.
10. Lozeron P, Lacour M-C, Vandendries C, et al. Contribution of plexus MRI in the diagnosis of atypical chronic inflammatory demyelinating polyneuropathies. J Neurol Sci 2016;360:170–5.
11. Nobile-Orazio E, Gallia F, Terenghi F, et al. Comparing treatment options for chronic inflammatory neuropathies and choosing the right treatment plan. Expert Rev Neurother 2017;17(8):755–65.
12. Van den Bergh PYK, Hadden RDM, Bouche P, et al. European Federation of Neurological Societies/Peripheral Nerve Society guideline on management of chronic inflammatory demyelinating polyradiculoneuropathy: report of a joint

task force of the European Federation of Neurological Societies and the Peripher. Eur J Neurol 2010;17(3):356–63.

13. Latov N, Deng C, Dalakas MC, et al. Timing and course of clinical response to intravenous immunoglobulin in chronic inflammatory demyelinating polyradiculo-neuropathy. Arch Neurol 2010;67(7):802–7.

14. Markvardsen LH, Sindrup SH, Christiansen I, et al. Subcutaneous immunoglob-ulin as first-line therapy in treatment-naive patients with chronic inflammatory demyelinating polyneuropathy: randomized controlled trial study. Eur J Neurol 2017;24(2):412–8.

15. van Schaik IN, Bril V, van Geloven N, et al. Subcutaneous immunoglobulin for maintenance treatment in chronic inflammatory demyelinating polyneuropathy (PATH): a randomised, double-blind, placebo-controlled, phase 3 trial. Lancet Neurol 2018;17(1):35–46.

16. Oaklander AL, Lunn MP, Hughes RA, et al. Treatments for chronic inflammatory demyelinating polyradiculoneuropathy (CIDP): an overview of systematic re-views. Cochrane Database Syst Rev 2017;(1):CD010369.

17. van Lieverloo GGA, Peric S, Doneddu PE, et al. Corticosteroids in chronic inflam-matory demyelinating polyneuropathy: a retrospective, multicentre study, comparing efficacy and safety of daily prednisolone, pulsed dexamethasone, and pulsed intravenous methylprednisolone. J Neurol 2018;265(9):2052–9.

18. Mahdi-Rogers M, Brassington R, Gunn AA, et al. Immunomodulatory treatment other than corticosteroids, immunoglobulin and plasma exchange for chronic in-flammatory demyelinating polyradiculoneuropathy. Cochrane Database Syst Rev 2017;(5):CD003280.

19. Dalakas MC. Advances in the diagnosis, immunopathogenesis and therapies of IgM-anti-MAG antibody-mediated neuropathies. Ther Adv Neurol Disord 2018; 11. 1756285617746640.

20. Dimachkie MM, Barohn RJ, Katz J. Multifocal motor neuropathy, multifocal ac-quired demyelinating sensory and motor neuropathy, and other chronic acquired demyelinating polyneuropathy variants. Neurol Clin 2013;31(2):533–55.

21. Bunschoten C, Jacobs BC, Van den Bergh PYK, et al. Progress in diagnosis and treatment of chronic inflammatory demyelinating polyradiculoneuropathy. Lancet Neurol 2019;18(8):784–94.

22. Yeh WZ, Dyck PJ, van den Berg LH, et al. Multifocal motor neuropathy: contro-versies and priorities. J Neurol Neurosurg Psychiatry 2019. https://doi.org/10. 1136/jnnp-2019-321532.

23. Willison HJ, Yuki N. Peripheral neuropathies and anti-glycolipid antibodies. Brain 2002;125(Pt 12):2591–625.

24. Querol L, Devaux J, Rojas-Garcia R, et al. Autoantibodies in chronic inflammatory neuropathies: diagnostic and therapeutic implications. Nat Rev Neurol 2017; 13(9):533–47.

25. Brannagan TH, Pradhan A, Heiman-Patterson T, et al. High-dose cyclophospha-mide without stem-cell rescue for refractory CIDP. Neurology 2002;58(12): 1856–8.

26. Vlam L, van der Pol W-L, Cats EA, et al. Multifocal motor neuropathy: diagnosis, pathogenesis and treatment strategies. Nat Rev Neurol 2011;8(1):48–58.

27. Beachy N, Satkowiak K, Gwathmey KG. Vasculitic neuropathies. Semin Neurol 2019;39(5):608–19.

28. Collins MP, Dyck PJB, Gronseth GS, et al. Peripheral Nerve Society Guideline on the classification, diagnosis, investigation, and immunosuppressive therapy of

non-systemic vasculitic neuropathy: executive summary. J Peripher Nerv Syst 2010;15(3):176–84.

29. Collins MP, Periquet MI, Mendell JR, et al. Nonsystemic vasculitic neuropathy: insights from a clinical cohort. Neurology 2003;61(5):623–30. Available at: http://www.ncbi.nlm.nih.gov/pubmed/12963752.

30. Zivković S a, Ascherman D, Lacomis D. Vasculitic neuropathy–electrodiagnostic findings and association with malignancies. Acta Neurol Scand 2007;115(6): 432–6.

31. Vrancken AFJE, Gathier CS, Cats EA, et al. The additional yield of combined nerve/muscle biopsy in vasculitic neuropathy. Eur J Neurol 2011;18(1):49–58.

32. Collins MP, Mendell JR, Periquet MI, et al. Superficial peroneal nerve/peroneus brevis muscle biopsy in vasculitic neuropathy. Neurology 2000;55(5):636–43. Available at: http://www.ncbi.nlm.nih.gov/pubmed/10980725.

33. Burns TM, Schaublin G a, Dyck PJB. Vasculitic neuropathies. Neurol Clin 2007; 25(1):89–113.

34. Gwathmey KG, Burns TM, Collins MP, et al. Vasculitic neuropathies. Lancet Neurol 2014;13(1):67–82.

35. Dyck PJ, Conn DL, Okazaki H. Necrotizing angiopathic neuropathy. Three-dimensional morphology of fiber degeneration related to sites of occluded vessels. Mayo Clin Proc 1972;47(7):461–75. Available at: http://www.ncbi.nlm.nih.gov/pubmed/4402730. Accessed April 7, 2013.

36. Nukada H, Dyck PJ. Microsphere embolization of nerve capillaries and fiber degeneration. Am J Pathol 1984;115(2):275–87. Available at: http://www.pubmedcentral.nih.gov/articlerender.fcgi?artid=1900501&tool=pmcentrez&rendertype=abstract. Accessed March 20, 2013.

37. Tracy J a, Engelstad JK, Dyck PJB. Microvasculitis in diabetic lumbosacral radiculoplexus neuropathy. J Clin Neuromuscul Dis 2009;11(1):44–8.

38. Nukada H, Dyck PJ, Karnes JL. Spatial distribution of capillaries in rat nerves: correlation to ischemic damage. Exp Neurol 1985;87(2):369–76. Available at: http://www.ncbi.nlm.nih.gov/pubmed/3967721. Accessed April 7, 2013.

39. Benstead TJ, Dyck PJ, Sangalang V. Inner perineurial cell vulnerability in ischemia. Brain Res 1989;489(1):177–81. Available at: http://www.ncbi.nlm.nih.gov/pubmed/2743147. Accessed April 7, 2013.

40. Collins MP, Periquet-Collins I, Sahenk Z, et al. Direct immunofluoresence in vasculitic neuropathy: specificity of vascular immune deposits. Muscle Nerve 2010; 42(1):62–9.

41. Said G, Lacroix C. Primary and secondary vasculitic neuropathy. J Neurol 2005; 252(6):633–41.

42. Schaublin G a, Michet CJ, Dyck PJB, et al. An update on the classification and treatment of vasculitic neuropathy. Lancet Neurol 2005;4(12):853–65.

43. Stone JH, Merkel P a, Spiera R, et al. Rituximab versus cyclophosphamide for ANCA-associated vasculitis. N Engl J Med 2010;363(3):221–32.

44. Fanouriakis A, Kougkas N, Vassilopoulos D, et al. Rituximab for eosinophilic granulomatosis with polyangiitis with severe vasculitic neuropathy: case report and review of current clinical evidence. Semin Arthritis Rheum 2015;45(1):60–6.

45. Jones RB, Tervaert JWC, Hauser T, et al. Rituximab versus cyclophosphamide in ANCA-associated renal vasculitis. N Engl J Med 2010;363(3):211–20.

46. Gold R, Fontana A, Zierz S. Therapy of neurological disorders in systemic vasculitis. Semin Neurol 2003;23(2):207–14.

47. Hoffman GS, Kerr GS, Leavitt RY, et al. Wegener granulomatosis: an analysis of 158 patients. Ann Intern Med 1992;116(6):488–98. Available at: http://www.ncbi.nlm.nih.gov/pubmed/1739240. Accessed August 23, 2013.

48. Gorson KC. Therapy for vasculitic neuropathies. Curr Treat Options Neurol 2006; 8(2):105–17. Available at: http://www.ncbi.nlm.nih.gov/pubmed/16464407. Accessed May 5, 2013.

49. Collins MP, Hadden RD. The nonsystemic vasculitic neuropathies. Nat Rev Neurol 2017;13(5):302–16.

50. Cacoub P, Terrier B, Saadoun D. Hepatitis C virus-induced vasculitis: therapeutic options. Ann Rheum Dis 2014;73(1):24–30.

51. Murai H, Inaba S, Kira J, et al. Hepatitis C virus associated cryoglobulinemic neuropathy successfully treated with plasma exchange. Artif Organs 1995;19(4): 334–8. Available at: http://www.ncbi.nlm.nih.gov/pubmed/7598653. Accessed April 9, 2013.

52. Scarpato S, Tirri E, Naclerio C, et al. Plasmapheresis in cryoglobulinemic neuropathy: a clinical study. Dig Liver Dis 2007;39(Suppl 1):S136–7. Available at: http://www.ncbi.nlm.nih.gov/pubmed/17936217. Accessed April 9, 2013.

53. Braun A, Neumann T, Oelzner P, et al. Cryoglobulinaemia type III with severe neuropathy and immune complex glomerulonephritis: remission after plasmapheresis and rituximab. Rheumatol Int 2008;28(5):503–6.

54. Ramos-Casals M, Stone JH, Cid MC, et al. The cryoglobulinaemias. Lancet 2012; 379(9813):348–60.

55. Montero N, Favà A, Rodriguez E, et al. Treatment for hepatitis C virus-associated mixed cryoglobulinaemia. Cochrane Database Syst Rev 2018;(5):CD011403.

56. Guillevin L, Lhote F, Leon A, et al. Treatment of polyarteritis nodosa related to hepatitis B virus with short term steroid therapy associated with antiviral agents and plasma exchanges. A prospective trial in 33 patients. J Rheumatol 1993;20(2): 289–98. Available at: http://www.ncbi.nlm.nih.gov/pubmed/8097249. Accessed April 9, 2013.

57. Teng GG, Chatham WW. Vasculitis related to viral and other microbial agents. Best Pract Res Clin Rheumatol 2015;29(2):226–43.

58. Dammacco F, Tucci FA, Lauletta G, et al. Pegylated interferon-alpha, ribavirin, and rituximab combined therapy of hepatitis C virus-related mixed cryoglobulinemia: a long-term study. Blood 2010;116(3):343–53.

59. Patel N, Patel N, Khan T, et al. HIV infection and clinical spectrum of associated vasculitides. Curr Rheumatol Rep 2011;13(6):506–12.

60. Wakasugi D, Kato T, Gono T, et al. Extreme efficacy of intravenous immunoglobulin therapy for severe burning pain in a patient with small fiber neuropathy associated with primary Sjögren's syndrome. Mod Rheumatol 2009;19(4):437–40.

61. Morozumi S, Kawagashira Y, Iijima M, et al. Intravenous immunoglobulin treatment for painful sensory neuropathy associated with Sjögren's syndrome. J Neurol Sci 2009;279(1–2):57–61.

62. McCoy SS, Baer AN. Neurological complications of Sjögren's syndrome: diagnosis and management. Curr Treat Options Rheumatol 2017;3(4):275–88.

63. Goodman BP. Immunoresponsive autonomic neuropathy in sjögren syndrome-case series and literature review. Am J Ther 2019;26(1):e66–71.

64. Alix JJP, Hadjivassiliou M, Ali R, et al. Sensory ganglionopathy with livedoid vasculopathy controlled by immunotherapy. Muscle Nerve 2015;51(2):296–301.

65. Gorson KC, Natarajan N, Ropper AH, et al. Rituximab treatment in patients with IVIg-dependent immune polyneuropathy: a prospective pilot trial. Muscle Nerve 2007;35(1):66–9.

66. Toledano P, Orueta R, Rodríguez-Pintó I, et al. Peripheral nervous system involvement in systemic lupus erythematosus: prevalence, clinical and immunological characteristics, treatment and outcome of a large cohort from a single centre. Autoimmun Rev 2017;16(7):750–5.

67. Fargetti S, Ugolini-Lopes MR, Pasoto SG, et al. Short- and long-term outcome of systemic lupus erythematosus peripheral neuropathy: bimodal pattern of onset and treatment response. J Clin Rheumatol 2019. https://doi.org/10.1097/RHU.0000000000001201.

68. Aletaha D, Neogi T, Silman AJ, et al. Rheumatoid arthritis classification criteria: an American College of Rheumatology/European League against Rheumatism collaborative initiative. Arthritis Rheum 2010;62(9):2569–81.

69. Puéchal X, Said G, Hilliquin P, et al. Peripheral neuropathy with necrotizing vasculitis in rheumatoid arthritis. A clinicopathologic and prognostic study of thirty-two patients. Arthritis Rheum 1995;38(11):1618–29. Available at: http://www.ncbi.nlm.nih.gov/pubmed/7488283. Accessed April 8, 2013.

70. Genta MS, Genta RM, Gabay C. Systemic rheumatoid vasculitis: a review. Semin Arthritis Rheum 2006;36(2):88–98.

71. Tavee JO, Karwa K, Ahmed Z, et al. Sarcoidosis-associated small fiber neuropathy in a large cohort: clinical aspects and response to IVIG and anti-TNF alpha treatment. Respir Med 2017;126:135–8.

72. Said G, Lacroix C, Planté-Bordeneuve V, et al. Nerve granulomas and vasculitis in sarcoid peripheral neuropathy. A clinicopathological study of 11 patients. Brain 2002;125(2):264–75.

73. Burns TM, Dyck PJB, Aksamit AJ, et al. The natural history and long-term outcome of 57 limb sarcoidosis neuropathy cases. J Neurol Sci 2006;244(1–2):77–87.

74. Fernandes SRM, Singsen BH, Hoffman GS. Sarcoidosis and systemic vasculitis. Semin Arthritis Rheum 2000;30(1):33–46.

75. Siva A, Saip S. The spectrum of nervous system involvement in Behçet's syndrome and its differential diagnosis. J Neurol 2009;256(4):513–29.

76. Tavee JO. Immune axonal polyneuropathy. Continuum (Minneap Minn) 2017;23(5, Peripheral Nerve and Motor Neuron Disorders):1394–410.

77. Ayrignac X, Viala K, Koutlidis RM, et al. Sensory chronic inflammatory demyelinating polyneuropathy: an under-recognized entity? Muscle Nerve 2013;48(5):727–32.

78. Nobile-Orazio E. Chronic inflammatory demyelinating polyradiculoneuropathy and variants: where we are and where we should go. J Peripher Nerv Syst 2014;19(1):2–13.

79. Eftimov F, van Schaik I. Chronic inflammatory demyelinating polyradiculoneuropathy: update on clinical features, phenotypes and treatment options. Curr Opin Neurol 2013;26(5):496–502.

80. Capasso M, Torrieri F, Di Muzio A, et al. Can electrophysiology differentiate polyneuropathy with anti-MAG/SGPG antibodies from chronic inflammatory demyelinating polyneuropathy? Clin Neurophysiol 2002;113(3):346–53.

81. Sinnreich M, Klein CJ, Daube JR, et al. Chronic immune sensory polyradiculopathy: a possibly treatable sensory ataxia. Neurology 2004;63(9):1662–9. Available at: http://www.ncbi.nlm.nih.gov/pubmed/15534252.

82. Collins MP, Periquet MI. Prevalence of vasculitic neuropathy in Wegener granulomatosis. Arch Neurol 2002;59(8):1333–4 [author reply: 1334]. Available at: http://www.ncbi.nlm.nih.gov/pubmed/12164733. Accessed May 4, 2013.

83. Comarmond C, Pagnoux C, Khellaf M, et al. Eosinophilic granulomatosis with polyangiitis (Churg-Strauss): clinical characteristics and long-term followup of the 383 patients enrolled in the French Vasculitis Study Group cohort. Arthritis Rheum 2013;65(1):270–81.

84. Moosig F, Bremer JP, Hellmich B, et al. A vasculitis centre based management strategy leads to improved outcome in eosinophilic granulomatosis and polyangiitis (Churg-Strauss, EGPA): monocentric experiences in 150 patients. Ann Rheum Dis 2012;1–7. https://doi.org/10.1136/annrheumdis-2012-201531.

85. Uchiyama M, Mitsuhashi Y, Yamazaki M, et al. Elderly cases of Churg-Strauss syndrome: case report and review of Japanese cases. J Dermatol 2012; 39(1):76–9.

86. Pagnoux C, Seror R, Henegar C, et al. Clinical features and outcomes in 348 patients with polyarteritis nodosa: a systematic retrospective study of patients diagnosed between 1963 and 2005 and entered into the French Vasculitis Study Group Database. Arthritis Rheum 2010;62(2):616–26.

87. Collins MP, Arnold WD, Kissel JT. The neuropathies of vasculitis. Neurol Clin 2013; 31(2):557–95.

88. Ferri C. Mixed cryoglobulinemia. Orphanet J Rare Dis 2008;3:25.

89. Saadoun D, Terrier B, Semoun O, et al. Hepatitis C virus-associated polyarteritis nodosa. Arthritis Care Res (Hoboken) 2011;63(3):427–35.

90. Ramos-Casals M, Robles A, Brito-Zerón P, et al. Life-threatening cryoglobulinemia: clinical and immunological characterization of 29 cases. Semin Arthritis Rheum 2006;36(3):189–96.

91. Migliaresi S, Di Iorio G, Ammendola A, et al. [Peripheral nervous system involvement in HCV-related mixed cryoglobulinemia]. Reumatismo 2001;53(1):26–32. Available at: http://www.ncbi.nlm.nih.gov/pubmed/12461575. Accessed May 2, 2013.

92. De Vita S, Quartuccio L, Isola M, et al. A randomized controlled trial of rituximab for the treatment of severe cryoglobulinemic vasculitis. Arthritis Rheum 2012; 64(3):843–53.

93. Grau RG. Drug-induced vasculitis: new insights and a changing lineup of suspects. Curr Rheumatol Rep 2015;17(12):71.

Immunotherapy for Peripheral Nerve Disorders

Andre Granger, MD, MBA, Elina Zakin, MD*

KEYWORDS

- Peripheral neuropathy • Corticosteroids • Prednisone • Methylprednisolone
- Immunoglobulin • Plasma exchange • Rituximab

KEY POINTS

- Immunosuppressive therapies are commonly used in the treatment of peripheral nerve disorders.
- In the geriatric population, these therapies require thoughtful decision making with careful attention to comorbid conditions and drug–drug interactions.
- Recommendations are provided for therapeutic agent selection, specific therapeutic dosing, laboratory monitoring, and other considerations.
- Therapeutic options presented include corticosteroids, immunoglobulin, plasma exchange, rituximab, and various steroid sparing agents, including mycophenolate mofetil, azathioprine, cyclophosphamide, and methotrexate.

INTRODUCTION

The peripheral nervous system serves motor, sensory, and autonomic functions. Thus, the symptoms that can be seen in these diseases can be highly variable and, at times, debilitating. Etiologies of peripheral nerve disorders can be divided into hereditary, inflammatory, paraneoplastic, metabolic, and toxic. Specifically, neuropathies mediated by inflammatory etiologies include acute or chronic inflammatory demyelinating polyradiculoneuropathy (CIDP), multifocal motor neuropathy, mononeuritis multiplex and neuropathy associated with connective tissue disorders. Although diabetes remains the most common cause of peripheral neuropathy in developed countries, these inflammatory conditions still account for a considerable number of nerve dysfunction disorders.[1]

Immunotherapy has been shown to significantly decrease, halt, and even reverse inflammatory peripheral nerve damage.[2] Corticosteroids are frequently used as a first-line therapeutic options in the management of peripheral neuropathies, especially

Department of Neurology, New York University Grossman School of Medicine, 660 1st Avenue, New York, NY 10016, USA
* Corresponding author.
E-mail address: Elina.zakin@nyulangone.org

Clin Geriatr Med 37 (2021) 347–359
https://doi.org/10.1016/j.cger.2021.01.007
0749-0690/21/© 2021 Elsevier Inc. All rights reserved.

geriatric.theclinics.com

early in the disease course or during exacerbations, owing their rapid onset of therapeutic efficacy, and large accessibility in comparison to other agent. The unfavorable side effect profile precludes prolonged use. This creates a role for steroid-sparing agents. Steroid-sparing agents including pharmacologic drugs rituximab, mycophenolate mofetil, cyclophosphamide, and azathioprine. Intravenous, as well as subcutaneous forms of immunoglobulin, have played a pivotal role in the management of neuroimmunologic disorders. In many cases in which immunoglobulin administration is being considered, therapeutic plasma exchange (TPE) may also be an option. Like all other groups of medications, anti-inflammatory treatments have various side effects. Selection of appropriate immunotherapy in the geriatric population requires special attention and should be patient specific.

PERIPHERAL NERVE DISORDERS TREATED WITH IMMUNOTHERAPY

Acute inflammatory demyelinating polyradiculoneuropathy and CIDP are typically characterized by progressive, ascending sensorimotor dysfunction and loss of deep tendon reflexes. They are further discussed in chapter 10 and 11 of this text. Multifocal motor neuropathy is a progressive, asymmetric, demyelinating lower motor neuron syndrome, usually affecting the distal limbs, also discussed in chapters 10 and 11 of this text. In mononeuritis multiplex, there is usually an underlying vasculitic process, and several separate peripheral nerves are affected in a stepwise manner. Patients usually report sensory and motor deficits that follow the distribution of specific nerves. Clinicians caring for patients with connective tissue disorders should be aware of the possible neurologic effects of this group of illnesses as vasculitic neuropathy is a common manifestation, and is further discussed in chapter 11 of this text.

GENERAL FACTORS TO CONSIDER WHEN CHOOSING AN AGENT

Several factors need to be considered when choosing treatment options in the geriatric patient population. As expected, older patients tend to have more comorbidities compared with younger patients. With increased comorbidities, there is a larger risk of developing polypharmacy and serious adverse events from drug interactions. Along with patient preferences, comorbidities may also affect decisions regarding routes of drug administration. Some patients may have illnesses that hinder oral medication administration or make intravenous access challenging.

Additional attention to the socioeconomic aspects of patient care is essential when selecting specific immunomodulatory therapy in geriatrics. The cost and availability of these medications should be thoroughly considered. For example, patients who need to receive infusions at specified centers should have a reliable and safe means to get to that location. Important consideration of the patient's baseline level of functioning should be taken into account when establishing reasonable therapeutic goals. This should also guide patient and family expectations. Life expectancy and goals of care need to be thoughtfully considered, especially if the patient is approaching the end of life. **Table 1** summarizes the key factors that should guide immunotherapy choice in the geriatric population.

Drug metabolism and excretion tend to slow down as patients age.[3] Additionally, the percentage of body weight composed of fat may also increase with age, and may also affect drug pharmacokinetics. These pharmacodynamic and pharmacokinetic factors may worsen the tolerance of medication adverse effects. In individuals with relapsing courses of illness, previously effective agents should be considered in the case of disease relapse.

Table 1	
Important factors affecting immunotherapy choices	
Patient's comorbidities	Prior therapeutic trials or interventions
Current medications	Drug pharmacokinetics
Drug route of administration	Patient's premorbid level of functioning
Drug side effect profile	Life expectancy
Patient tolerance	Goals of care
Drug availability and cost	Level of distress that symptoms cause
Time for drug to reach peak efficacy	Drug interactions

Immunization schedule deserves attention before initiation of immunotherapy. Live vaccines should be given 2 to 4 weeks ahead of immunomodulating therapy. Inactivated vaccines, can be given, but efficacy may be decreased. Thus, vaccine administration 2 to 4 weeks before treatment may be more beneficial. In patients 50 years or older, 2 doses of inactivated zoster vaccine, separated by 2 to 6 months, are advised (if not previously given). Regardless of the point in the treatment protocol, inactivated influenza vaccine should be administered every flu season, annually. Pneumococcal vaccine recommendations vary depending on age. If under 65 years, 1 dose of conjugate vaccine, followed by 2 doses polysaccharide vaccine (at $\geq$8 weeks and at $\geq$5 years from first dose). If 65 years or older, the polysaccharide vaccine should be given at least 1 year after the conjugate vaccine.[4]

FREQUENTLY USED IMMUNOTHERAPIES IN PERIPHERAL NERVE DISORDERS
Corticosteroids

Corticosteroids belong to a group of medications that mimic the function of adrenal hormones. They achieve their immunomodulatory effects through decreasing the function and migration of immune cells.[5] Prednisone and methylprednisolone are commonly used drugs for the treatment of peripheral nerve disorders in this category. Prednisone is administered orally, whereas methylprednisolone can be given orally or intravenously. Prednisone is readily absorbed from the gastrointestinal tract and has a bioavailability of 60% to 100%, but this can be altered in individuals with hepatic failure, chronic renal failure, inflammatory bowel disease, and hyperthyroidism. It is converted to its active form, prednisolone, by the liver. Its half-life is 2 to 3 hours, with a time to peak with the immediate release formulation of 2 hours. It is excreted in the urine. Methylprednisolone has an onset of action of 1 hour, peaks in about 2.1 hours, and has a half-life of 2.5 hours. It is metabolized by the liver and excreted in the urine.[6–10] Only the methylprednisolone succinate formulation, also known as Solu-Medrol can be given intravenously. Initial high-dose pulse therapy should be considered for neuropathies secondary to specific severe systemic rheumatologic disorders with typical weight-based dosing of 7 to 15 mg/kg per dose (typically 500 mg to 1 g), administered daily for 3 to 5 days. **Table 2** provides an overview of typical immunosuppression agents and their dosages used for specific peripheral nerve diseases.

The side effect profile of corticosteroids calls for careful analysis before administration in the geriatric patient. In fact, it is recommended that, if they are needed, they should be used for the shortest possible time and at the lowest possible dose. Oral prednisone dosing of 1 mg/kg daily is advised at therapeutic initiation (60 mg/d for most adults). Intravenous pulse doses can also be considered at initiation (500 mg to 1 g daily) for 3 to 5 days, with subsequent switch to 1 mg/kg oral dosing daily.

Table 2
Common peripheral nerve disorders with recommended immunotherapy

Peripheral Nerve Disorder	Commonly Used Immunotherapy
AIDP	IVIg: 2 g/kg usually divided over 5 d TPE: usually 5–7 sessions; volume of plasma exchanged calculated based on patient's height, weight, sex, and hematocrit
CIDP	IVIg: typically 1 mg/kg, given over 2–3 d on a monthly basis (depending on clinical course) TPE: biweekly initially then based on patient's response Prednisone: 60–80 mg/d for 2–3 mo, then slow taper by 10 mg weekly, or gradual replacement with steroid sparing agent Mycophenolate mofetil: 500 mg twice daily initial dose; increase based on response and tolerability to a maintenance dose of 1.0 g to 1.5 g twice daily. May be added as monotherapy or in conjunction with glucocorticoids. Azathioprine: 50 mg/d initial dose, increase by 50 mg increments every 1–2 wk to a target dose of 2.5–3 mg/kg/d. May be added as monotherapy or in conjunction with glucocorticoids Cyclophosphamide (IV): 1 g/m² every 4 wk
Multifocal motor neuropathy	IVIg: typically 1 mg/kg, given over 2–3 d on a monthly basis (depending on clinical course) Cyclophosphamide (IV): 1 g/m² every 4 wk
Mononeuritis multiplex	Treatment varies; treat based on underlying disorder – usually vasculitis. Corticosteroids useful.
PND associated with CTD	Treatment varies; can be guided by standard of care for the underlying CTD

Abbreviations: AIDP, acute inflammatory demyelinating polyradiculoneuropathy; CTD, connective tissue diseases; IV, intravenous; IVIg, intravenous immunoglobulin; PND, peripheral nerve disorders.
Data from Refs.[4,16,24]

The tapering of oral prednisone therapy should be slow, especially in cases of CIDP or vasculitic neuropathy, often by 5 to 10 mg every 2 weeks from an initial dose of more than 40 mg/d. The goal of tapering is to use a rate of change that will prevent both recurrent activity of the disease and symptoms of cortisol deficiency owing to persistent hypothalamic–pituitary axis suppression. Monitoring for patient response is critical as the taper continues. At doses of prednisone that are less than 5 mg/d, there is a decreased likelihood of hypothalamic–pituitary axis suppression. If prolonged therapy with oral corticosteroids is poorly tolerated, an alternative approach of interval dosing of intravenous pulse doses of methylprednisolone could be considered (ie, 3–5 days of 500 mg to 1 g of intravenous methylprednisolone every 2–4 weeks). Studies have demonstrated no difference between the various dosing schedules and modes of administration in terms of efficacy and safety.

The more common or concerning risk factors for prolonged corticosteroid administration include behavioral changes, sleep disturbances, fluid retention, weight gain, Cushing's syndrome, insulin insensitivity, gastrointestinal ulceration, infection, aseptic necrosis of the femoral or humeral head, osteoporosis, and glaucoma. They should be used with caution if the patient is also taking mineralocorticoids, loop or thiazide diuretics, other immunosuppressants, nonsteroidal anti-inflammatory drugs, warfarin, or CYP3A4 inducers or inhibitors.[11] Shorter courses are favored, and slow tapers are recommended for courses of longer than 7 to 10 days. In cases of vasculitic neuropathy, a very slow course of steroid taper should be performed (as noted elsewhere in this article). In such cases, early initiation of steroid-sparing agents are alternatives to prolonged steroid regimens, usually at the start of the prolonged steroid taper, because the onset of action of the steroid-sparing agents may be 6 to 12 months from initiation of dosing. For steroid courses expected to be administered for more than 4 weeks, prophylaxis against *Pneumocystis jirovecii* pneumonia with oral trimethoprim/sulfamethoxazole, and supplementation of calcium and vitamin D, should be initiated. Doses of trimethoprim/sulfamethoxazole studied and most often used are double strength 800 mg/160 mg once daily, administered 3 times weekly.[12] **Table 3** provides a list of key factors that should be monitored in geriatric patients prescribed immune-modulating therapies.

Mycophenolate Mofetil

Mycophenolate mofetil is an inhibitor of inosine monophosphate dehydrogenase, which results in decreased B- and T-cell function through the inhibition of de novo guanosine synthesis. It is completely metabolized in the liver to its active metabolite and excreted as metabolites in the urine. The oral tablet possesses a bioavailability of about 90% and a half-life of about 16 hours. Time to peak is about 1 to 2 hours.[13] The therapeutic efficacy of mycophenolate mofetil administration usually takes 6 to 12 months to achieve, so it is important to initiate therapy early in the course of disease when decision for prolonged steroid use (>4 weeks) is made. Mycophenolate mofetil is used in the treatment of CIDP and vasculitic neuropathies.

Patients with severe renal disease should be monitored for dose-dependent adverse effects. A complete blood count should be checked weekly for the first month, twice monthly during months 2 to 5, and monthly for the remainder of the first year. Liver function tests should also be monitored monthly. Skin cancer screening should be performed annually, given the increased risk of systemic malignancy. Clinicians should monitor for signs and symptoms of infection.[14]

Azathioprine

Azathioprine is a mercaptopurine derivative whose metabolite is incorporated into DNA, eventually halting purine synthesis.[15] It is metabolized in the liver and excreted as inactive metabolites in the urine. Indications for use of azathioprine include CIDP, multifocal motor neuropathy, and vasculitic neuropathy associated with connective tissue diseases. Initial dose is oral 50 mg/d with increase of 50 mg every 1 to 2 weeks, until the target dose of 2.5 to 3.0 mg/kg/d. Azathioprine can be used as monotherapy or in conjunction with a corticosteroid. This medication is associated with bone marrow toxicity, infection, malignancy, nausea, vomiting, hepatotoxicity, and myalgia. A complete blood count as well as liver and renal function tests should be checked weekly on initiation for 1 month, then every 2 weeks for 2 months, followed by twice annually.[16] It is recommended that patients be checked for thiopurine S-methyltransferase gene mutations because this may help to identify patients at higher risk of severe adverse reactions (bone marrow suppression).[17] Skin cancer screening should be performed annually, given increased risk of systemic malignancy.

Cyclophosphamide

Cyclophosphamide crosslinks DNA leading to decreased DNA synthesis and cell replication. It is metabolized in the liver to active metabolites.[18] The literature has

Table 3
Important considerations for monitoring on immunomodulatory therapy

Therapy	Laboratory Monitoring	Other Monitoring	Special Considerations
Corticosteroids	Hemoglobin A1c before starting. Electrolytes and blood glucose within 2 wk of initiating, then every 3–6 mo. Check hepatitis panel and tuberculin skin test/interferon gamma release assay before infusion. Screen for HIV if ≤65 y, or increased risk (eg, sexual or intravenous drug use exposure)	Ophthalmology examination at 6 wk, then annually for glaucoma and cataracts. Blood pressure at initiation then at least twice per year. For those taking ≥2.5 mg prednisone daily for ≥3 mo, bone density testing within 6 mo of starting treatment for patients >40 years old, then every 1–3 y on treatment is recommended. For Fracture Risk Assessment Tool score ≥10% (moderate or high fracture risk), initiate bisphosphonates	If taking ≥20 mg of prednisone daily for ≥1 mo with another immunosuppressant or ≥30 mg/d for ≥1 mo, then administer TMP-SMX 160–800 mg/d or 3 d per week, or TMP-SMX 80/400 mg/d. For courses ≥1 mo, add 1000–1200 mg calcium and 600–800 units of vitamin D daily. Lifestyle modifications (quitting smoking, alcohol use reduction, weight bearing exercise, maintenance of weight in normal range).
IVIg	Check renal function and CBC at initiation then every 3–6 mo. Check IgA levels before starting.	Monitor vitals during infusions.	Acetaminophen 650 mg, ibuprofen 400–600 mg, and/or diphenhydramine 25 mg can be used (with caution in the elderly) to decreased adverse reactions, administered as pretreatment.
TPE	Check coagulation factors (including fibrinogen) and electrolytes (including calcium and potassium) before first session and after each session.	Monitor vitals during exchanges.	Calcium gluconate 1000 mg should be ordered with each exchange session to maintain a normal calcium level.
Rituximab	Check hepatitis panel and tuberculin skin test/interferon gamma release assay before infusion. If Hepatitis B core antibody present, then check hepatitis B PCR every 6 mo. Check JC virus antibody before infusion Monitor CBC and immunoglobulins before each session.	Check vital signs during each session. Check electrocardiogram during infusion in patients with cardiac comorbidities. Serum lymphocyte subset analysis (with attention to CD20+ B cells) can be performed to assess drug effect.	

Mycophenolate mofetil	Monitor CBC with differential and complete metabolic panel every week for the first month, every 2 wk for months 2–5, and monthly for the remainder of the first year. Check LFTs monthly.	Skin cancer screening annually
Azathioprine	Check for TPMT mutation before initiation. Weekly CBC with differential, creatinine, LFT ×4 weeks, then every 2 wk × 2 mo, then twice annually. Check hepatitis panel and tuberculin skin test/interferon gamma release assay before infusion.	Skin cancer screening annually
Cyclophosphamide	CBC with differential, urinalysis, and complete metabolic panels should be monitored every 6 mo.	Check urinalysis if patient has urinary complaints (evaluation for hemorrhagic cystitis).
Methotrexate	CBC, complete metabolic panels every month for 2 mo, then twice annually. Check chest radiographs and pulmonary function tests if signs of toxicity develop or at least annually.	Check methotrexate level if signs of toxicity develop.

Abbreviations: CBC, complete blood count; GI, gastrointestinal; HIV, human immunodeficiency virus; IgA, immunoglobulin A; IVIg, intravenous immunoglobulin; LFT, liver function tests; TB, tuberculosis; TMP-SMX, Trimethoprim-sulfamethoxazole; TPMT, thiopurine S-methyltransferase.
Data from Refs.[4,24,30,32]

demonstrated a role for cyclophosphamide in CIDP, multifocal motor neuropathy, and mononeuritis multiplex.[19] The modes of administration include oral and intravenous. Oral dosing is recommended at 1.5 to 3.0 mg/kg per day. Intravenous dosing is performed as pulse dose 1 g/m^2 every 4 weeks.[4] Bone marrow suppression, infection, and gastrointestinal symptoms can be experienced by some patients. Patients should also be monitored for hemorrhagic cystitis and cardiopulmonary toxicity. Blood count and a urinalysis, along with liver and renal function panels, should be included in follow-up analyses, and checked every 6 months.

Methotrexate

Through the inhibition of dihydrofolate reductase, methotrexate hinders DNA synthesis and cellular replication. Metabolism occurs partially in the gut, then in the liver. Despite the lack of high-quality evidence, there have been a few cases of CIDP that showed good response to methotrexate.[20,21] Methotrexate has been investigated as an alternative for patients on chronic intravenous immunoglobulin (IVIg) with mixed results in 1 study.[22] Methotrexate is usually administered orally, with dosing at 5 mg weekly on initiation. Dose increase is performed slowly, typically 2.5 mg per week, to a goal of 25 mg weekly. In individuals who are unable to tolerate oral administration, typically owing to gastrointestinal side effects, the same oral weekly dose may be administered subcutaneously or intramuscularly. Thrombotic events, diabetes mellitus, bone marrow suppression, elevated liver enzymes, infection, and pulmonary disease are among the adverse effects of the drug. A complete blood count, comprehensive metabolic panels, and methotrexate levels should be monitored monthly for the first 2 months of therapy, then twice annually thereafter. Additional surveillance for pulmonary fibrosis with chest radiographs and pulmonary function tests should be performed annually.[23]

Intravenous Immunoglobulins

Therapeutic immune globulin is a preparation of polyclonal IgG acquired from several blood or plasma donors.[24] Its first licensed use in the United States dates back to the early 1980s.[25] Although it has been in use for some time, the exact mechanism of action remains unclear. Theories include interference with both the variable and constant regions of IgG antibodies, interaction with their target receptors, competition with pathologic autoantibodies, and upregulation of inhibitory immune mechanisms.[24] Intramuscular, subcutaneous, and intravenous formulations are available, with the intravenous preparation being the most commonly used. The initial therapeutic response may be seen in the first several days, and effects last up to 3 to 4 weeks with intravenous and intramuscular formulations. The half-life is about 23 days if administered intramuscularly, about 59 days if administered subcutaneously, and 14 to 24 days if administered intravenously.[24,26]

The typical loading dose of IVIg is 2 g/kg divided into 2 to 5 daily doses.[24] The maintenance dose of IVIg is typically 1 mg/kg, given over 2 to 3 days every 4 weeks (depending on the clinical course). Drug levels are not monitored, but renal function, as well as hemoglobin and hematocrit, should be followed. Adverse reactions are typically minor, although serious morbidity can ensue. Early adverse effects include headaches, fever, chills, and myalgias.[24] Preceding treatment with analgesics, nonsteroidal anti-inflammatory drugs, antihistamines, and, less commonly, glucocorticoids may decrease the risk of adverse reactions.[27] In patients deficient in IgA, there is an increased risk of anaphylactic reactions. As such, it is important to check serum IgA levels before the initiation of immunoglobulin therapy. In patients with low serum IgA levels, the use of formulations with lower IgA content is advised. Late effects are rare, but are particularly important in the elderly, who may already be at increased risk for these complications. They include acute renal failure and thrombotic events. Advanced age, previous thrombotic disease, diabetes mellitus, dehydration, immobility, and nephrotoxic medications can increase these risks. Thromboembolic complications may be increased in patients concurrently receiving estrogen therapy. IVIg may also decrease the efficacy of some live vaccines.[27]

Therapeutic Plasma Exchange

TPE, also called plasmapheresis, was first used therapeutically in 1952 in a patient with hyperviscosity owing to a primary blood disorder.[28] This therapeutic procedure involves exchange of the patient's plasma with an isosmotic replacement fluid, usually 5% albumin, via automated, extracorporeal machinery. Its effect is thought to be achieved through the replacement of pathogenic autoantibodies, immune complexes, and cytokines.[29] The use of TPE requires trained individuals and specific equipment, which can limit its use in some settings. Its onset of action is relatively rapid, but the time to noticeable recovery varies based on the disease being treated and the specific course in the individual disease process. Calculations of volume of plasma to be removed are based on the patient's height, weight, sex, and hematocrit. This procedure requires the placement of a vascular access that permits high blood flow. Endogenous serum immunoglobulin levels decrease to 40% to 60% of baseline after 2 sessions of TPE. For neurologic causes, induction therapy with a cycle of treatment typically consists of 5 to 7 exchange sessions, each occurring every other day.[29] Results can be short lived and repeat cycles of therapy can be administered on a weekly, biweekly, or monthly schedule.

As mentioned elsewhere in this article, the use of TPE requires the placement of a large-bore intravenous catheter. Furthermore, most of the complications associated with TPE are related to line placement, fluid disequilibrium, and the removal of useful macromolecules. Potential complications related to central line placement include infection, bleeding, hematoma formation, neurovascular damage, thrombosis, air emboli, and pneumothoraxes. Hypotension and its related complications can occur during TPE sessions.[30] Roughly 200 mL of the patient's blood can remain within the tubing and other parts of the machine. Some patients, such as those with low blood volumes, cardiac disease, or neurovascular stenosis, may be more sensitive to these changes in volume, making this therapeutic modality more concerning for use in the geriatric patient population. Decreasing flow rates during the procedure may dampen these effects.

The choice of replacement fluid influences the effect of macromolecule removal. If fresh frozen plasma is used over albumin, there will be a smaller coagulation factor deficit. However, the use of albumin decreases the possibility of severe allergic reactions. Citrate is used as an anticoagulant in the TPE system and can lead to hypocalcemia. Reduction in potassium, coagulation factors, immunoglobulins, and highly protein-bound medications may occur.[30] The case fatality rate has been reported to be 3 to 5 per 10,000.[31] Before the first session, the patient's risk of complications should be estimated, and a coagulation panel and fibrinogen should be checked. These tests should also be repeated every 1 to 2 days and corrective action taken if deranged. Calcium replacement is usually routinely ordered with each session.

Rituximab

Rituximab is a chimeric monoclonal antibody against the B-cell surface marker CD20. The variable portion of rituximab binds to the CD20 surface marker, whereas the constant portion initiates immune responses that eventually lead to the destruction of about 90% of circulating B-cells within 3 days of infusion. The half-life ranges from approximately 10 to 30 days. B-cell depletion lasts for at least 6 months in most patients.[32] In patients with peripheral nerve disorders that are refractory to first-line therapies, such as immunoglobulin, corticosteroid, or plasma exchange, consideration of rituximab is appropriate.

Rituximab confers a higher risk of myocardial infarction, pulmonary events, arrhythmia, and acutely worsening severe cardiac failure in elderly patients at risk. Additionally, owing to its immunosuppressive effects, clinicians should be aware of the patient's hepatitis B, hepatitis C, and tuberculosis status, with the greatest risk seen with hepatitis B.[32] Other noteworthy risks include infusion reactions (highest risk with first infusion), mucocutaneous reactions (including Stevens–Johnson syndrome), hepatobiliary disease, infection, secondary antibody deficiency, neutropenia, progressive multifocal leukoencephalopathy, and posterior reversible encephalopathy syndrome.[32] Rituximab should be used with extreme caution in patients on other immunosuppressants. Live immunizations should not be administered before or during rituximab therapy. Inactivated vaccines should be given 4 weeks or more before therapy.[33] Complete blood counts with differential and platelets should be obtained at least before each treatment. Electrolytes and renal function should also be monitored before each treatment. Vital signs must be watched closely during each infusion. Cardiac monitoring is recommended in the elderly, especially those with preexisting cardiac disease. Serum lymphocyte subset analysis may be performed, with attention to CD20+ subset several months after therapy, as there are large intraindividual variations of B-cell repopulation. The literature suggests that higher body surface area correlates to early B-cell repopulation, with therapeutic drug efficacy as low as 3.6 months.[34–42]

SUMMARY

The geriatric population is a unique group and requires special consideration in the management of immune-mediated peripheral nerve disorders. Each immunotherapeutic option has a potential for various adverse effects; therefore, a careful assessment of each agent should be performed, with therapy tailored to each patient. Corticosteroids, IVIgs, and TPE are the most commonly used immune-modulating agents. All clinicians who see geriatric patients should be aware of the acute and delayed effects of these modalities in this specific patient population, especially those taking multiple medications or who have numerous comorbidities. It is also important to consider the side effect profiles of the various steroid-sparing agents available when making a selection for the geriatric patient who requires prolonged courses of corticosteroid administration.

CLINICS CARE POINTS

- Geriatric patients' goals of care, comorbidities, and drug side effect profile should be considered when choosing a therapeutic agent.
- Corticosteroids, effective in therapy for both CIDP and mononeuritis multiplex, require additional monitoring of serum glucose, blood pressure, and bone density and are often preferred owing to their rapid efficacy of action.
- In addition to immune suppression, common side effects of prolonged corticosteroid therapy include osteoporosis, weight gain, hyperglycemia, skin changes, and possible steroid-mediated psychosis.

- Long standing corticosteroid use requires prophylaxis against *Pneumocystis jirovecii* pneumonia with trimethoprim/sulfamethoxazole, and supplementation of calcium and vitamin D.

- IVIg requires intravenous administration and should be used with caution in individuals with history of thrombotic events.

- Plasma exchange requires central venous access and further monitoring for dilutional coagulopathy, and may result in hemodynamic fluctuations, an important factor to consider with use in the elderly.

- The use of steroid-sparing agents, including azathioprine, cyclophosphamide, mycophenolate mofetil, and rituximab, requires further monitoring of complete blood counts and comprehensive metabolic panels

DISCLOSURE

The authors have nothing to disclose.

REFERENCES

1. Hanewinckel R, Ikram MA, Van Doorn PA. Peripheral neuropathies. Handb Clin Neurol 2016;138:263–82.
2. Muley SA, Parry GJ. Inflammatory demyelinating neuropathies. Curr Treat Options Neurol 2009;11(3):221–7.
3. Klotz U. Pharmacokinetics and drug metabolism in the elderly. Drug Metab Rev 2009;41(2):67–76.
4. Cartwright SL, Cartwright MS. Health maintenance for adults with neuromuscular diseases on immunosuppression. Muscle Nerve 2019;59(4):397–403.
5. Lester RS. Corticosteroids. Clin Dermatol 1989;7(3):80–97.
6. Frey BM, Frey FJ. Clinical pharmacokinetics of prednisone and prednisolone. Clin Pharmacokinet 1990;19(2):126–46.
7. Czock D, Keller F, Rasche FM, et al. Pharmacokinetics and pharmacodynamics of systemically administered glucocorticoids. Clin Pharmacokinet 2005;44(1):61–98.
8. Gambertoglio JG, Amend WJ Jr, Benet LZ. Pharmacokinetics and bioavailability of prednisone and prednisolone in healthy volunteers and patients: a review. J Pharmacokinet Biopharm 1980;8(1):1–52.
9. Hughes RA, Mehndiratta MM, Rajabally YA. Corticosteroids for chronic inflammatory demyelinating polyradiculoneuropathy. Cochrane Database Syst Rev 2017;(11):CD002062.
10. Van den Bergh PY, Rajabally YA. Chronic inflammatory demyelinating polyradiculoneuropathy. Presse Med 2013;42(6 Pt 2):e203–15.
11. Buchman AL. Side effects of corticosteroid therapy. J Clin Gastroenterol 2001;33(4):289–94.
12. Park JW, Curtis JR, Moon J, et al. Prophylactic effect of trimethoprim-sulfamethoxazole for pneumocystis pneumonia in patients with rheumatic diseases exposed to prolonged high-dose glucocorticoids. Ann Rheum Dis 2018;77(5):644–9.
13. Bullingham RE, Nicholls AJ, Kamm BR. Clinical pharmacokinetics of mycophenolate mofetil. Clin Pharmacokinet 1998;34(6):429–55.
14. Elimelakh M, Dayton V, Park KS, et al. Red cell aplasia and autoimmune hemolytic anemia following immunosuppression with alemtuzumab, mycophenolate, and

daclizumab in pancreas transplant recipients. Haematologica 2007;92(8): 1029–36.

15. Taylor AL, Watson CJ, Bradley JA. Immunosuppressive agents in solid organ transplantation: mechanisms of action and therapeutic efficacy. Crit Rev Oncol Hematol 2005;56(1):23–46.

16. American College of Rheumatology Subcommittee on Rheumatoid Arthritis Group. Guidelines for the management of rheumatoid arthritis: 2002 update. Arthritis Rheum 2002;46(2):328–46.

17. Relling MV, Gardner EE, Sandborn WJ, et al. Clinical pharmacogenetics implementation consortium guidelines for thiopurine methyltransferase genotype and thiopurine dosing: 2013 update. Clin Pharmacol Ther 2013;93(4):324–5.

18. Emadi A, Jones RJ, Brodsky RA. Cyclophosphamide and cancer: golden anniversary. Nat Rev Clin Oncol 2009;6(11):638–47.

19. Niermeijer JM, Eurelings M, van der Linden MW, et al. Intermittent cyclophosphamide with prednisone versus placebo for polyneuropathy with IgM monoclonal gammopathy. Neurology 2007;69(1):50–9.

20. Group RMCT. Randomised controlled trial of methotrexate for chronic inflammatory demyelinating polyradiculoneuropathy (RMC trial): a pilot, multicentre study. Lancet Neurol 2009;8(2):158–64.

21. Diaz-Manera J, Rojas-Garcia R, Gallardo E, et al. Response to methotrexate in a chronic inflammatory demyelinating polyradiculoneuropathy patient. Muscle Nerve 2009;39(3):386–8.

22. Nobile-Orazio E, Terenghi F, Cocito D, et al. Oral methotrexate as adjunctive therapy in patients with multifocal motor neuropathy on chronic IVIg therapy. J Peripher Nerv Syst 2009;14(3):203–5.

23. Karadag AS, Kanbay A, Ozlu E, et al. Pulmonary fibrosis developed secondary to methotrexate use in a patient with psoriasis vulgaris. North Clin Istanb 2015;2(2): 159–61.

24. Lunemann JD, Nimmerjahn F, Dalakas MC. Intravenous immunoglobulin in neurology–mode of action and clinical efficacy. Nat Rev Neurol 2015;11(2):80–9.

25. Younger DS. Peripheral nerve disorders. Prim Care 2004;31(1):67–83.

26. Koleba T, Ensom MH. Pharmacokinetics of intravenous immunoglobulin: a systematic review. Pharmacotherapy 2006;26(6):813–27.

27. Orbach H, Katz U, Sherer Y, et al. Intravenous immunoglobulin: adverse effects and safe administration. Clin Rev Allergy Immunol 2005;29(3):173–84.

28. Adams WS, Blahd WH, Bassett SH. A method of human plasmapheresis. Proc Soc Exp Biol Med 1952;80(2):377–9.

29. Lehmann HC, Hartung HP. Plasma exchange and intravenous immunoglobulins: mechanism of action in immune-mediated neuropathies. J Neuroimmunol 2011; 231(1–2):61–9.

30. Michaud D, McKay L, Pfefferle P, et al. Therapeutic plasma exchange. Dynamics 2001;12(4):18–24.

31. Mokrzycki MH, Kaplan AA. Therapeutic plasma exchange: complications and management. Am J Kidney Dis 1994;23(6):817–27.

32. Whittam DH, Tallantyre EC, Jolles S, et al. Rituximab in neurological disease: principles, evidence and practice. Pract Neurol 2019;19(1):5–20.

33. Friedman MA, Winthrop KL. Vaccines and disease-modifying antirheumatic drugs: practical implications for the rheumatologist. Rheum Dis Clin North Am 2017;43(1):1–13.

34. Ellwardt E, Ellwardt L, Bittner S, et al. Monitoring B-cell repopulation after depletion therapy in neurologic patients. Neurol Neuroimmunol Neuroinflamm 2018; 5(4):e463.

35. van der Meche FG, Schmitz PI. A randomized trial comparing intravenous immune globulin and plasma exchange in Guillain-Barre syndrome. Dutch Guillain-Barre Study Group. N Engl J Med 1992;326(17):1123–9.

36. Randomised trial of plasma exchange, intravenous immunoglobulin, and combined treatments in Guillain-Barre syndrome. Plasma Exchange/Sandoglobulin Guillain-Barre Syndrome Trial Group. Lancet 1997;349(9047):225–30.

37. Hughes RA, Donofrio P, Bril V, et al. Intravenous immune globulin (10% caprylate-chromatography purified) for the treatment of chronic inflammatory demyelinating polyradiculoneuropathy (ICE study): a randomised placebo-controlled trial. Lancet Neurol 2008;7(2):136–44.

38. Nobile-Orazio E, Cocito D, Jann S, et al. Intravenous immunoglobulin versus intravenous methylprednisolone for chronic inflammatory demyelinating polyradiculoneuropathy: a randomised controlled trial. Lancet Neurol 2012;11(6): 493–502.

39. van Schaik IN, Bril V, van Geloven N, et al. Subcutaneous immunoglobulin for maintenance treatment in chronic inflammatory demyelinating polyneuropathy (PATH): a randomised, double-blind, placebo-controlled, phase 3 trial. Lancet Neurol 2018;17(1):35–46.

40. Hahn AF, Bolton CF, Zochodne D, et al. Intravenous immunoglobulin treatment in chronic inflammatory demyelinating polyneuropathy. A double-blind, placebo-controlled, cross-over study. Brain 1996;119(Pt 4):1067–77.

41. Dyck PJ, Litchy WJ, Kratz KM, et al. A plasma exchange versus immune globulin infusion trial in chronic inflammatory demyelinating polyradiculoneuropathy. Ann Neurol 1994;36(6):838–45.

42. Lehmann HC, Hoffmann FR, Fusshoeller A, et al. The clinical value of therapeutic plasma exchange in multifocal motor neuropathy. J Neurol Sci 2008; 271(1–2):34–9.

Management of Neuropathic Pain in the Geriatric Population

Elizabeth J. Pedowitz, MD[a],*, Rory M.C. Abrams, MD[b],
David M. Simpson, MD[c]

KEYWORDS

- Neuropathic pain • Neuropathy • Geriatrics • Elderly • Management • Treatment

KEY POINTS

- Neuropathic pain is common and a major cause of morbidity and suffering in the geriatric population.
- It is important to differentiate neuropathic pain from other types of pain, as the treatment options are different than those used for nociceptive or visceral pain.
- Clinicians must take greater caution in treating neuropathic pain in the elderly to avoid drug-drug interactions and iatrogenic effects of medications.
- Alternative nonmedication therapies and topical treatments should be considered given the lack of systemic effects.
- When systemic medications are needed, initiate with monotherapy at lowest possible doses and titrate up slowly while monitoring closely for adverse effects.

INTRODUCTION

The International Association for the Study of Pain defines neuropathic pain as pain caused by a lesion or disease of the somatosensory nervous system.[1] Older adults are at an increased risk of neuropathic pain because many diseases that cause neuropathy increase in incidence with age. These include diabetes (diabetic neuropathy), herpes zoster (postherpetic neuralgia), spinal degenerative disease, radiculopathies, many cancers and associated chemotherapy use, stroke (central neuropathic pain), and limb amputations (phantom limb pain).[2] Other common causes of neuropathy include vitamin deficiencies, alcohol abuse, and human immunodeficiency virus (HIV).[3] There are limited

[a] Brookdale Department of Geriatrics and Palliative Medicine, Icahn School of Medicine at Mount Sinai, 1468 Madison Avenue, Annenberg, 10th Floor, New York, NY 10029, USA; [b] Department of Neurology, Division of Neuromuscular Diseases and Clinical Neurophysiology Laboratories, Icahn School of Medicine at Mount Sinai, 1000 Tenth Avenue, 10th Floor Suite 10C, New York, NY 10019, USA; [c] Department of Neurology Division of Neuromuscular Diseases and Clinical Neurophysiology Laboratories, Icahn School of Medicine at Mount Sinai, 1468 Madison Avenue, Annenberg, 2nd Floor, Box 1052, New York, NY 10029, USA
* Corresponding author.
E-mail address: Elizabeth.Pedowitz@mssm.edu

Clin Geriatr Med 37 (2021) 361–376
https://doi.org/10.1016/j.cger.2021.01.008
0749-0690/21/© 2021 Elsevier Inc. All rights reserved.

data on the prevalence of neuropathic pain in the elderly population, although some reports indicate a prevalence of up to 32%.[4–6] Despite neuropathic pain being common and representing a major cause of morbidity and suffering in the elderly population, older adults are underrepresented in clinical trials of medications for neuropathic pain, making it difficult to generalize the benefits and risks of treatment of older individuals.[2]

CLINICAL FEATURES OF NEUROPATHIC PAIN AND DISTINGUISHING FROM OTHER TYPES OF PAIN

Neuropathic pain is characterized by several symptoms and signs. Neuropathic pain classically has a burning, electrical, or sharp quality. Unlike nociceptive pain, patients will also often have other associated "positive" symptoms such as tingling, prickling, and skin tightening sensations along with "negative" symptoms such as numbness, loss of sensation, and a "falling asleep" sensation.[7] Furthermore, patients with neuropathic pain will often have neurologic examination findings consistent with a peripheral neuropathy syndrome such as distal symmetric polyneuropathy, pure small fiber neuropathy, and compression mononeuropathy (see chapter in this issue titled, "A clinical approach to disease of peripheral nerve"). Outside of peripheral neuropathy, several other neurologic diseases are associated with neuropathic pain. These diseases include cervical and lumbar radiculopathy, herpes zoster, trigeminal neuralgia, poststroke pain, and postspinal cord injury pain.[8]

DIAGNOSIS OF NEUROPATHIC PAIN

The clinical features of neuropathic pain and neuropathy form the groundwork for diagnosis. There are screening tools such as the Neuropathic Pain Scale and the Neuropathic Pain Questionnaire that can aid in diagnosis and quantification of severity.[9,10] These scales, however, fail to identify 10% to 20% of patients with neuropathic pain, so they are no substitute for careful clinical assessment.[11]

Although self-reporting is considered the gold standard for evaluating pain, older adults may have difficulties communicating about their pain for a variety of reasons including cognitive impairment and language dysfunction.[12] Any acute change of behavior in the elderly, especially those with difficulties communicating, should prompt providers to consider pain as a potential cause. It may be important to obtain collateral information from family members about the patient's expression of pain. There are also behavioral scales for pain evaluation in elderly patients with communication disorders such as Algoplus and Doloplus, although these were not specifically developed for neuropathic pain.[5,13–15] These observational scales, especially for patients with dementia, focus on facial expressions, body language, and vocalizations.[16] It is also important to recognize that a relationship exists between the effects of neuropathic pain on mood and sleep dysfunction.[17] A study of patients aged 65 years and older with postherpetic neuralgia found that the pain interfered most with general activity, mood, sleep, and enjoyment of life.[18] Another study in patients with painful diabetic neuropathy with a mean age of 61 years reported that more than 60% reported moderate or severe interference with general activity, mood, walking ability, normal work, sleep, and enjoyment of life.[19] The presence of mood and sleep disorders should prompt a consideration into searching for provoking causes of pain including peripheral neuropathy. There can be a relationship between conditions such as anxiety or depression and pain, and managing these psychological comorbidities is important.[20] In a study examining predictors of new-onset distal neuropathic pain in HIV-infected individuals, older age and more severe depression both conferred a significant risk.[21]

Patients with suspected neuropathic pain should also be evaluated for other associated findings of peripheral neuropathy. The evaluation of patients with suspected peripheral neuropathy via physical examination, laboratory testing, electrodiagnostic testing, and nerve biopsy is covered in other articles in this series.

TREATMENT

Treatment of neuropathic pain focuses on identifying and treating reversible causes (if any) while simultaneously providing symptom management. It is important that clinicians and patients understand that providing disease-specific therapy does not necessarily mean resolution of symptoms. For example, this may be the case with diabetes where chronic axonal changes are slow to resolve or may even be irreversible.[22] Furthermore, most patients do not achieve complete pain relief with symptomatic treatment but can expect the pain to be more tolerable.[20] Improvement in patient's function and quality of life is paramount rather than eradication of pain, which is often not possible. For these reasons, it is important to set realistic expectations of treatment goals with patients and explain that predicting treatment response is difficult and there is sometimes a trial and error period.

Each geriatric patient must be treated individually in the context of their clinical situation, comorbidities, metabolic function, other medications, and cognitive status. Given multiple comorbidities, polypharmacy, and physiologic changes affecting drug metabolism are all common in the geriatric population, the risk of iatrogenic disease and serious drug-drug interactions are high.[5] Studies evaluating drugs for neuropathic pain are limited in the elderly population, and randomized controlled trials often exclude elderly patients.[23] It is advisable to initiate with monotherapy at the lowest possible doses with slow upward titration to analgesic effect while monitoring for adverse effects.[5,6,24] The risks and benefits of each medication must be considered in each patient, and interval monitoring for adverse reactions and efficacy should be planned.[25] **Table 1** contains a list of pharmacologic therapies in the elderly with starting doses, suggested dose increment, typical dose, and potential adverse effects. Clinicians should frequently reassess how the neuropathic pain affects the patient's quality of life, activities of daily living, and functional status.[26]

Most randomized controlled drug trials in neuropathic pain have been for limited indications. The US Food and Drug Administration (FDA) has approved 6 medications for 3 neuropathic pain syndromes: painful diabetic neuropathy (pregabalin, duloxetine, and capsaicin 8% patch), postherpetic neuralgia (gabapentin, pregabalin, 5% lidocaine patch, capsaicin cream, and capsaicin 8% patch), and trigeminal neuralgia (carbamazepine).[20] Non-FDA approved medications have also been found to be effective in clinical practice.[27] The current National Institute for Health and Care Excellence guidance for the pharmaceutical management of neuropathic pain suggests offering a choice of amitriptyline, duloxetine, gabapentin, or pregabalin as initial treatment of neuropathic pain (with the exception of trigeminal neuralgia) and switching if the first, second, or third drugs are not effective or tolerated.[28] This concurs with other recent guidelines from the Neuropathic Pain Special Interest Group (NeuPSIG) of the International Association for the Study of Pain, which has gabapentin, pregabalin, serotonin-norepinephrine reuptake inhibitors (SNRIs; duloxetine/venlafaxine), and tricyclic antidepressants (TCAs) as first-line agents and capsaicin 8% patches, lidocaine patches, and tramadol as second-line agents.[27] In frail and elderly patients, lidocaine patches may be considered as a first-line agent.[27]

PHARMACOLOGIC OPTIONS
Calcium Channel α2-δ Ligands (Gabapentin/Pregabalin)

Gabapentinoids are a first-line class of medications in the treatment of neuropathic pain.[11,29,30] They bind to the voltage-gated calcium channels at the α2-δ subunit

Table 1
Pharmacologic therapies for neuropathic pain in the elderly

Drug Class	Agent	Route	Initial Dose	Dose Increment	Typical Dose	Adverse Effects
Calcium Channel α2-δ Ligands	Gabapentin	PO	100–300 mg daily three times/d	100–300mg daily in 1-3 divided doses	300-2700mg daily in 1-3 divided doses	• Sedation, altered mental status • Dizziness, ataxia • Visual disturbances • Peripheral edema; recommend caution with heart failure • Administer at lower doses in renal failure to avoid excess sedation, dizziness
	Pregabalin	PO	25–75 mg daily three times/d	25–75mg daily in 1-3 divided doses	50-300mg daily in 2-3 divided doses	
Serotonin-Norepinephrine Reuptake Inhibitors	Duloxetine	PO	20–30 mg daily	Increase 20–30 mg every 1 wk	60 mg daily	• Sedation • Nausea, constipation • Dry mouth • Hypertension, palpitations • Caution with cardiac conduction derangements • Taper on cessation to avoid withdrawal syndrome
	Venlafaxine	PO	37.5 mg daily	37.5–75 mg every 1-2 wk	150–225 mg daily (extended release)	

Drug Class	Drug	Route	Starting Dose	Titration	Maximum Dose	Side Effects/Cautions
Tricyclic Antidepressants	Amitriptyline Desipramine Nortriptyline	PO	10–20 mg daily	Increase 10–25 mg every 1 wk	25–75 mg daily	• Fewer anticholinergic effects with nortriptyline: sedation, dizziness, falls, dry mouth, constipation, urinary retention • Caution with cardiovascular disease and cardiac conduction derangements • Avoid in glaucoma, prostate hypertrophy, angina, heart failure, cardiac conduction abnormalities
Alpha Lipoic Acid		IV/PO	600 mg		600–1800 mg daily	• Nausea and vomiting
Cannabinoids		INH/PO				• Sedation • Dizziness • Confusion/psychosis • Abuse potential
Sodium Channel Antagonists	Carbamazepine	PO	100–200 mg daily	100–200mg/day every 1 wk	600–800mg/day in 3–4 divided doses	• Sedation • Dizziness • Skin rash • Rarely, can cause hyponatremia, leukopenia, thrombocytopenia, and liver damage

(continued on next page)

Table 1
(continued)

Drug Class	Agent	Route	Initial Dose	Dose Increment	Typical Dose	Adverse Effects
Topical Agents	Lidocaine patch 4 or 5%	Topical	1–4 patches daily for maximum 12 h			• Local skin irritation, redness, rash • Erythema, burning, and pain at application site • Consider topical pretreatment with lidocaine and oral analgesics before application
	Capsaicin patch/cream	Topical	0.075% (low-dose cream)/8% (high-dose patch)			

and produce changes in neurotransmitter release.[31] They have an overall better safety profile than many other oral therapeutic options, with few drug-drug interactions due to their lack of metabolism or effect on hepatic enzymes. However, they can cause adverse effects such as sedation, dizziness, ataxia, visual disturbances, altered mental status, or peripheral edema.[32] Patients with chronic kidney disease and especially those on hemodialysis are more susceptible to complications due to reduced clearance of these agents, as they depend on renal excretion for elimination.[33] Clinical guidelines recommend conservative dosing of gabapentin and pregabalin, up to a maximum dose of 300 mg or 100 mg daily, respectively, for treatment of neuropathic pain in those with end-stage renal disease.[33]

A Cochrane review found moderate-quality evidence that oral gabapentin has an important effect on pain in some people with moderate or severe neuropathic pain after shingles or due to diabetes.[34] Typical starting dose of gabapentin is 100 to 300 mg three times a day with titration every 1 to 7 days by 100 to 300 mg/d as tolerated up to a maximum dose of 3600 mg/d[20] To reduce daytime side effects including sedation, providers may start with a single bedtime dose; this may also be a favorable strategy when the pain is most bothersome at night. There may be a delayed onset to reach analgesic effect, taking up to 2 months.[8] Elderly patients should be started on the lowest dose (100 mg at bedtime) and titrated up slowly assessing for adverse effects.[25]

A Cochrane review found moderate-quality evidence that oral pregabalin has an important effect on pain in some people with moderate or severe neuropathic pain after shingles or due to diabetes.[35] Pregabalin doses start at 150 mg/d divided in 2 to 3 doses with titration every 1 to 2 weeks to a maximum dose of 300 mg/d[8] However, older adults should be started at low doses (50 mg at bedtime) and titrated up slowly to assess tolerance.[25] It should be used cautiously in patients with heart failure, because cases of decompensated heart failure with pregabalin use have been reported.[3]

Serotonin-Norepinephrine Reuptake Inhibitors

SNRIs, such as duloxetine and venlafaxine, regulate descending inhibitory pathways of pain via inhibition of serotonin and norepinephrine reuptake. SNRIs can also be used for treatment of comorbid depression and anxiety.[36] SNRIs have a better safety profile than TCAs, but there are still many potential adverse effects in the elderly including nausea, constipation, hot flashes, hyperhidrosis, palpitations, dry mouth, hypertension, and drug-drug interactions including a risk of serotonergic syndrome.

Duloxetine is considered a first-line neuropathic agent.[11,27,28] Duloxetine has a single daily dosing regimen and also acts as an antidepressant. It has been found to be effective in maintaining pain relief for 6 months in an open-label trial in patients with painful diabetic neuropathy.[37] Older adults should be started at 20 to 30 mg once daily and after 1 week can be increased to 60 mg once daily as tolerated.[23,25]

Venlafaxine is used in the treatment of major depressive disorder and generalized anxiety disorder, social anxiety disorder, panic disorder, and agoraphobia. A Cochrane review evaluating venlafaxine in neuropathic pain found that there is an inadequate amount of information available to promote it as a first-line agent for neuropathic pain but that it is a reasonably well-tolerated drug and may be of some benefit in patients not able to tolerate other drugs.[38] If it is to be started, it should be at a low dose of 37.5 mg daily and blood pressure and heart rate should be monitored.[25] It should not be abruptly stopped, as there can be a withdrawal syndrome.[20]

Tricyclic Antidepressants

TCAs, such as amitriptyline, are often considered first-line medications for treating neuropathic pain. They work by inhibiting the reuptake of serotonin and norepinephrine and blocking ion channels, which reinforces the descending inhibitory pain pathways.[36,39] They should, however, be used with significant caution in the geriatric population. The anticholinergic adverse effects may be significant in elderly patients and can provoke dizziness, sedation, orthostatic hypotension, dry mouth, and constipation. They are contraindicated in patients with glaucoma, prostate hypertrophy, or certain cardiac conditions including unstable angina, recent myocardial infarction, heart failure, and abnormal cardiac conduction. They can also contribute to cognitive disorders or confusion. Because of this risk profile, other neuropathic agents may be preferable in the geriatric population.[40] Tertiary amine TCAs such as amitriptyline, imipramine, and clomipramine are not recommended at doses greater than 75 mg/d in older adults because of major anticholinergic and sedative side effects and potential risk of falls.[27] Nortriptyline is a secondary amine TCA that has fewer anticholinergic side effects, but a Cochrane review found little evidence to support the use of nortriptyline to treat neuropathic pain.[41]

Carbamazepine

Carbamazepine is approved by the FDA for treatment of trigeminal neuralgia, which is a specific form of neuropathic pain that is not fully covered in this article but deserves mention. A Cochrane review in 2014 found that it is also probably effective in some people with chronic neuropathic pain but with reservations given the lack of trial evidence.[42] The drug is a sodium channel antagonist and works by slowing the recovery rate of the voltage-gated sodium channels.[8] The precise mechanism of action in relation to relief of neuropathic pain remains uncertain, but they reduce the ability of the neuron to fire at high frequency and likely inhibits ectopic discharges.[42,43] Side effects include drowsiness, difficulties with balance, skin rash, and dizziness. Rarer severe side effects include agranulocytosis, thrombocytopenia, and liver damage. Regular monitoring with complete blood count and liver function testing is recommended. There is a high potential for drug-drug interactions, as carbamazepine is an inducer of the hepatic P450 cytochrome system. It also has a narrow therapeutic window.[44] Dosing guidelines suggest starting at 200 to 400 mg/d in 2 to 4 divided doses per day depending on preparation and gradually increasing over several weeks in increments of 100 to 200 mg every 2 days as needed. The usual maintenance dose is 600 to 800 mg/d with a maximum dose of 1,200 mg/d. In chronic therapy, it should be withdrawn gradually over 2 to 6 months to minimize withdrawal symptoms.[45] Therapeutic drug monitoring may be useful, especially within the first few months of therapy, as carbamazepine induces hepatic enzymes, thereby increasing its own metabolism. It should be used with caution in the elderly population, especially given the significant drug interactions and the need for laboratory monitoring with its use.

Opioids

Opioids are considered second- or third-line agents in the treatment of neuropathic pain. Systematic review and meta-analyses find opioids do provide analgesic effect in neuropathic pain in the short term (the average duration of treatment in trials was 5 weeks with a range of 1–16 weeks), although little is known about long-term efficacy.[27,46] There are significant safety concerns including opioid abuse and addiction in patients suffering from chronic pain. Every patient should be assessed for risk factors related to potential abuse and strictly monitored. The lowest effective dose should be prescribed. Opioids should only be used in certain situations with severe, refractory pain such as during titration of a first-line medication, acute exacerbations of chronic neuropathic pain, or in the setting of malignancy.[8]

Constipation, somnolence, delirium, dizziness, nausea, and dry mouth are the most commonly reported adverse effects of opioids.[47] Respiratory depression is one of the major concerns of opioid therapy, especially in patients also using benzodiazepines or barbiturates.[48] Patients generally develop tolerance to all of the adverse effects except constipation, and it is important that a bowel regimen is started with initiation of opioids.

Tramadol is a weak opioid that acts as both mu-opioid agonist and norepinephrine and serotonin reuptake inhibitor. It has a similar side effect profile to other opioids. It also lowers the seizure threshold and can cause serotonin syndrome if combined with other selective serotonin reuptake inhibitors. Doses should be reduced in elderly patients and in those with renal or hepatic impairment.[49] A Cochrane review found only low- or very low–quality evidence and was unable to make a conclusion about its efficacy and safety in treating neuropathic pain.[49,50]

Strong opioids include morphine, hydromorphone, oxycodone, and fentanyl. Caution should be used in the elderly given the increased half-life of the active drug metabolites and especially if there is hepatic or renal failure.[27] When considering use of opioids to control neuropathic pain, it may be most appropriate to refer to a pain management specialist.

Alpha Lipoic Acid

Alpha lipoic acid (ALA) is an antioxidant substance that has been studied in the treatment of neuropathic pain, specifically in diabetic peripheral neuropathy (DPN). It is thought to relieve pain by reducing oxidative stress, which is an important mechanism in the pathogenesis of diabetic peripheral neuropathy.[49] Based on a 2012 meta-analysis, ALA, 600 mg, administered intravenously daily for 3 weeks led to a clinically significant reduction in neuropathic pain in the short term.[51] A randomized, double-blind, placebo-controlled trial demonstrated oral treatment with ALA, 600 mg, daily for 5 weeks improved neuropathic symptoms in those with distal symmetric polyneuropathy, and a prospective, double-blinded, placebo-controlled study demonstrated oral 600 mg ALA twice daily for DPN over 6 months is effective, safe, and tolerable.[52,53] There is currently a Cochrane review pending to assess the effects of ALA as a disease-modifying agent in DPN.[54] Relative to other treatments for peripheral neuropathy, there are fewer side effects, although it can cause nausea and vomiting.[49]

Topical Treatments

Topical medications with their limited systemic effects warrant special consideration in the elderly population who often have multiple comorbidities and polypharmacy. They are especially useful in localized neuropathic pain where the area of maximum pain is consistent and circumscribed. A review article evaluated topical treatment of localized neuropathic pain in the elderly, including 18 randomized controlled trials. It determined that in older adults, lidocaine 5% and capsaicin 8% are effective for localized neuropathic pain and considered first-line drugs in older adults, especially in patients with comorbidities and polypharmacy.[55,56]

Lidocaine is a local anesthetic available in plaster (patch), spray, or cream that acts as a sodium-channel antagonist, and acts to reduce ectopic discharges mediating nociception.[36,55] The 4% lidocaine patch is sold over-the-counter, whereas the 5% patch requires a prescription in the United States. Both strengths of patches have the same administration guidelines and can be self-applied facilitating patient adherence.[55] Side effects are rare and are largely related to local skin reactions. Clinical experience and individual studies indicate it is effective for pain relief in older persons, although the Cochrane review in adults found no evidence from good-quality randomized controlled trials to support its use.[57] Topical lidocaine can also be used in combination with an oral neuropathic pain medication. One study found combination of lidocaine 5% medicated plaster with pregabalin provided additional relief from pain due to postherpetic neuralgia and diabetic polyneuropathy and was safe and well tolerated.[58] The American Geriatrics Society states that all patients with localized neuropathic pain are candidates for topical lidocaine (moderate quality of evidence, strong recommendation).[25]

Capsaicin is the active ingredient of chili peppers. It binds to nociceptors in the skin, specifically the transient receptor potential vanilloid 1 receptor. Following continued capsaicin exposure, there is reversible degeneration of the nerve terminals preventing pain transmission and resulting in a reduced pain response.[8,55] A Cochrane review found there is moderate-quality evidence that high-concentration (8%) capsaicin patches can give moderate pain relief or better to a minority of people with postherpetic neuralgia and very low–quality evidence that it benefits those with HIV neuropathy and diabetic neuropathy.[59] One study found that the capsaicin 8% patch is noninferior to an optimized dose of pregabalin in relieving pain in patients with peripheral neuropathic pain with a more rapid onset of action, fewer systemic side effects, and greater treatment satisfaction.[60] Another randomized, double-blind, placebo-controlled study found that one 30-minute treatment with the capsaicin 8% patch provided modest improvements in pain and sleep quality in patients with painful diabetic peripheral neuropathy.[61] The high-concentration patch is applied by a physician for 30 to 60 minutes and may provide relief for up to 12 weeks.[55] It may require pretreatment with topical lidocaine or oral analgesia due to the intense pain with initial application, with some patients even experiencing an increase in blood pressure during the painful application. Some adverse effects include local erythema, edema, and swelling and sensory complaints of burning or stinging pain. It can cause mucous membrane irritation and must be handled by the provider and patient with caution.[8] In spite of these adverse effects, a double-blind study in patients with diabetes found the treatment to be well tolerated with no discontinuations due to drug-related reactions.[61]

ALTERNATIVE TREATMENTS
Movement and Physical Therapy

Physical therapy can help improve functionality and mobility, which is important, as neuropathy often leads to a decrease in physical activity. A focus on strengthening muscles and improving balance are crucial to successful physical therapy for neuropathy.[8] The effects of exercise may even reduce inflammation. Studies have demonstrated improvement in cutaneous nerve regeneration capacity in patients with metabolic syndrome and diabetes who undergo exercise regimens, specifically moderate intensity aerobic exercise for 150 minutes a week.[62,63] In patients with diabetic neuropathy, physical movement helps improve glycemic control, which can prevent worsening of the neuropathy.[64]

Tai chi and yoga are other types of physical engagement that have proved beneficial in ameliorating various chronic pain conditions. Tai chi is a traditional Chinese martial art consisting of low-impact, low-velocity smooth movements to improve balance, prevent falls, enhance cardiovascular health, and reduce stress. Twelve weeks of Tai chi (1 hour, 3 times per week) improved fasting blood glucose, insulin resistance, hemoglobin A1c, balance, and Total Symptom Score in diabetic neuropathy in 2 controlled trials.[65,66] Yoga has been shown to be beneficial in neurologic disorders, pain, and diabetes in multiple studies, but randomized controlled trials in neuropathy are limited.[67,68] A randomized controlled trial showed superiority of the practice of yoga postures compared with splinting in treatment of carpal tunnel syndrome for improvement in pain and grip strength.[69]

Psychotherapy

Cognitive behavioral therapy (CBT) aids patients in changing maladaptive behaviors, thoughts, and emotions by teaching coping skills and conscious confrontation of deleterious thoughts and behaviors.[64] CBT has been shown to provide benefit in patients with HIV-related peripheral neuropathy, improving pain and reducing pain-related interference with functioning in these patients.[70] A Cochrane review found insufficient evidence of the efficacy of psychological interventions for neuropathic pain given the lack of studies specifically examining this.[71] However, a study of 442 patients with chronic pain comparing the use of telephone CBT, exercise, or a combination of both showed significantly better outcomes for the combined intervention group at 6 and 9 months.[72]

There are a few studies demonstrating a benefit of other integrative psychotherapies in reducing pain and improving quality of life. Specifically, self-hypnosis was found to be useful and well tolerated in a small group of patients with HIV-related distal sensory polyneuropathy.[73] Mindfulness meditation and progressive relaxation meditation were found to be beneficial as part of a comprehensive pain management plan for older adults with painful diabetic neuropathy in 2 small studies.[74,75] However, other studies have not shown a statistically significant change on pain and quality of life with meditation in patients with neuropathic pain.[76,77]

Acupuncture

Acupuncture involves stimulation of anatomic points through solid metallic needle penetration and manipulation. It is a therapy based on traditional Chinese medicine. A systematic review and meta-analysis of acupuncture for the treatment of peripheral neuropathy showed benefit for acupuncture over control in the treatment of diabetic neuropathy and probable benefit for treatment of HIV-related neuropathy. The study concluded that more rigorously designed studies are needed using sham acupuncture.[78] However, a Cochrane review found insufficient evidence to support or refuse the use of acupuncture in treating neuropathic pain, given the studies were small and of low-quality evidence with limited generalizability.[79]

Cannabinoids

The role of cannabis-based medicines in treating neuropathic pain is controversial. A Cochrane review demonstrated a lack of high-quality evidence that any cannabis-derived product works for chronic neuropathic pain but that the potential benefits of cannabis-based medicine in chronic neuropathic pain might be outweighed by their potential harms.[80] A randomized, double-blind, placebo-controlled crossover study done in 16 patients with painful diabetic peripheral neuropathy assessing the short-term efficacy and tolerability of inhaled cannabis demonstrated a dose-dependent reduction in diabetic peripheral neuropathic pain.[81] Possible side effects include sedation, dizziness, and confusion, and its use is limited by availability, abuse potential, and the risk of precipitating psychosis.[8] Cannabinoids have a weak recommendation against their use in neuropathic pain by the NeuPSIG based on their systematic review.[27]

SUMMARY

Neuropathic pain can be challenging to diagnose and treat, especially in elderly patients. It is important to correctly diagnose neuropathic pain and evaluate possible causes, of which there are many. Pharmacologic treatments should be prescribed cautiously given the increased risk of side effects in the geriatric population. However, it is important to not let caution impede adequate pain control. For localized pain, topical treatments should be considered. Nonpharmacologic alternative treatments should be considered as additive therapy. Frequent reevaluation to assess for analgesic effect and potential adverse events is important.

CLINICS CARE POINTS

- Neuropathic pain is common and a major cause of morbidity and suffering in the geriatric population.
- Neuropathic pain can be difficult to distinguish from other types of pain, and diagnosis requires a thorough history and physical examination.
- Referral to a neurologist and nerve conduction studies and electromyography may be required.
- Once diagnosed, further workup is required to elucidate the cause, including potential reversible causes of neuropathy.
- Symptoms of neuropathic pain can be "positive" such as burning or tingling or "negative" such as numbness.
- Pharmacologic treatments can often improve the "positive" symptoms, but it is difficult to treat the "negative" symptoms.
- It is important to differentiate neuropathic pain from other types of pain, as the treatment options are quite different than those used for nociceptive or visceral pain.
- Older adults are underrepresented in clinical trials of medications for neuropathic pain, making it difficult to generalize the benefits and risks of treatment in older individuals.
- Clinicians must take greater caution in treating neuropathic pain in the elderly to avoid drug-drug interactions and iatrogenic effects of medications.
- Alternative nonmedication therapies and topical treatments should be considered.
- When systemic medications are needed, initiate with monotherapy at lowest possible doses and titrate up slowly while monitoring closely for adverse effects.
- It is important to not be overcautious at the risk of undertreating patients' pain. Risks and benefits must be considered and frequent reevaluation is necessary.

DISCLOSURE

The authors have nothing to disclose.

REFERENCES

1. Treede R-D, Jensen TS, Campbell JN, et al. Neuropathic pain: redefinition and a grading system for clinical and research purposes. Neurology 2008;70(18): 1630–5.
2. Schmader KE, Baron R, Haanpää ML, et al. Treatment considerations for elderly and frail patients with neuropathic pain. Mayo Clin Proc 2010;85(3 Suppl): S26–32.
3. Snyder MJ, Gibbs LM, Lindsay TJ. Treating painful diabetic peripheral neuropathy: an update. Am Fam Physician 2016;94(3):227–34.
4. Stompór M, Grodzicki T, Stompór T, et al. Prevalence of chronic pain, particularly with neuropathic component, and its effect on overall functioning of elderly patients. Med Sci Monit Int Med J Exp Clin Res 2019;25:2695–701.

5. Pickering G, Marcoux M, Chapiro S, et al. An Algorithm for neuropathic pain management in older people. Drugs Aging 2016;33(8):575–83.
6. Pickering G. Analgesic use in the older person. Curr Opin Support Palliat Care 2012;6(2):207–12.
7. Gierthmühlen J, Baron R. Neuropathic pain. Semin Neurol 2016;36(5):462–8.
8. Zakin E, Simpson D. Neuropathic pain. In: Nair KPS, González-Fernández M, Panicker JN, editors. Neurorehabilitation therapy and therapeutics. New York: Cambridge University Press; 2018. p. 144–57.
9. Krause SJ, Backonja M-M. Development of a neuropathic pain questionnaire. Clin J Pain 2003;19(5):306–14.
10. Galer BS, Jensen MP. Development and preliminary validation of a pain measure specific to neuropathic pain: the Neuropathic Pain Scale. Neurology 1997;48(2):332–8.
11. Cruccu G, Sommer C, Anand P, et al. EFNS guidelines on neuropathic pain assessment: revised 2009. Eur J Neurol 2010;17(8):1010–8.
12. Tracy B, Sean Morrison R. Pain management in older adults. Clin Ther 2013;35(11):1659–68.
13. Rat P, Jouve E, Pickering G, et al. Validation of an acute pain-behavior scale for older persons with inability to communicate verbally: Algoplus. Eur J Pain Lond Engl 2011;15(2):198.e1-10.
14. Rostad HM, Utne I, Grov EK, et al. Measurement properties, feasibility and clinical utility of the Doloplus-2 pain scale in older adults with cognitive impairment: a systematic review. BMC Geriatr 2017;17(1):257.
15. Wary B, Doloplus C. [Doloplus-2, a scale for pain measurement]. Soins Gerontol 1999;(19):25–7.
16. Savvas SM, Gibson SJ. Overview of pain management in older adults. Clin Geriatr Med 2016;32(4):635–50.
17. Vinik A. The approach to the management of the patient with neuropathic pain. J Clin Endocrinol Metab 2010;95(11):4802–11.
18. Oster G, Harding G, Dukes E, et al. Pain, medication use, and health-related quality of life in older persons with postherpetic neuralgia: results from a population-based survey. J Pain 2005;6(6):356–63.
19. Gore M, Brandenburg NA, Dukes E, et al. Pain severity in diabetic peripheral neuropathy is associated with patient functioning, symptom levels of anxiety and depression, and sleep. J Pain Symptom Manage 2005;30(4):374–85.
20. Zilliox LA. Neuropathic pain. Contin Lifelong Learn Neurol 2017;23(2):512.
21. Malvar J, Vaida F, Sanders CF, et al. Predictors of new-onset distal neuropathic pain in HIV-infected individuals in the era of combination antiretroviral therapy. Pain 2015;156(4):731–9.
22. Rogers LC, Frykberg RG, Armstrong DG, et al. The Charcot foot in diabetes. Diabetes Care 2011;34(9):2123–9.
23. Chai E, Horton JR. Managing pain in the elderly population: Pearls and Pitfalls. Curr Pain Headache Rep 2010;14(6):409–17.
24. Makris UE, Abrams RC, Gurland B, et al. Management of persistent pain in the older patient: a clinical review. JAMA 2014;312(8):825–36.
25. American geriatrics Society Panel on the pharmacological management of persistent pain in older persons. Pharmacological management of persistent pain in older persons. Pain Med Malden Mass 2009;10(6):1062–83.
26. Fine PG. Treatment guidelines for the pharmacological management of pain in older persons. Pain Med Malden Mass 2012;13(Suppl 2):S57–66.

27. Finnerup NB, Attal N, Haroutounian S, et al. Pharmacotherapy for neuropathic pain in adults: a systematic review and meta-analysis. Lancet Neurol 2015; 14(2):162–73.
28. Overview | Neuropathic pain in adults: pharmacological management in non-specialist settings | Guidance | NICE. Available at: https://www.nice.org.uk/guidance/cg173. Accessed April 6, 2020.
29. Bril V, England JD, Franklin GM, et al. Evidence-based guideline: treatment of painful diabetic neuropathy–report of the American association of neuromuscular and electrodiagnostic medicine, the American Academy of Neurology, and the American Academy of physical medicine & Rehabilitation. Muscle Nerve 2011; 43(6):910–7.
30. Verma V, Singh N, Singh Jaggi A. Pregabalin in neuropathic pain: evidences and possible mechanisms. Curr Neuropharmacol 2014;12(1):44–56.
31. Kremer M, Salvat E, Muller A, et al. Antidepressants and gabapentinoids in neuropathic pain: Mechanistic insights. Neuroscience 2016;338:183–206.
32. Onakpoya IJ, Thomas ET, Lee JJ, et al. Benefits and harms of pregabalin in the management of neuropathic pain: a rapid review and meta-analysis of randomised clinical trials. BMJ Open 2019;9(1):e023600.
33. Ishida JH, McCulloch CE, Steinman MA, et al. Gabapentin and pregabalin Use and association with adverse outcomes among hemodialysis patients. J Am Soc Nephrol JASN 2018;29(7):1970–8.
34. Wiffen PJ, Derry S, Bell RF, et al. Gabapentin for chronic neuropathic pain in adults. Cochrane Database Syst Rev 2017;(6):CD007938.
35. Derry S, Bell R, Straube S, et al. Pregabalin for neuropathic pain in adults. Cochrane Database Syst Rev 2019;(1):CD007076.
36. Zakin E, Abrams R, Simpson DM. Diabetic neuropathy. Semin Neurol 2019; 39(05):560–9.
37. Raskin J, Wang F, Pritchett YL, et al. Duloxetine for patients with diabetic peripheral neuropathic pain: a 6-month open-label safety study. Pain Med 2006;7(5): 373–85.
38. Gallagher HC, Gallagher RM, Butler M, et al. Venlafaxine for neuropathic pain in adults. Cochrane Database Syst Rev 2015;(8):CD011091.
39. Bravo L, Llorca-Torralba M, Berrocoso E, et al. Monoamines as drug targets in chronic pain: focusing on neuropathic pain. Front Neurosci 2019;13. https://doi.org/10.3389/fnins.2019.01268.
40. Cruccu G, Truini A. A review of neuropathic pain: from guidelines to clinical practice. Pain Ther 2017;6(1):35–42.
41. Derry S, Wiffen PJ, Aldington D, et al. Nortriptyline for neuropathic pain in adults. Cochrane Database Syst Rev 2015;(1):CD011209.
42. Wiffen PJ, Derry S, Moore RA, et al. Carbamazepine for chronic neuropathic pain and fibromyalgia in adults. Cochrane Database Syst Rev 2014;4. https://doi.org/10.1002/14651858.CD005451.pub3.
43. Tremont-Lukats IW, Megeff C, Backonja MM. Anticonvulsants for neuropathic pain syndromes: mechanisms of action and place in therapy. Drugs 2000; 60(5):1029–52.
44. Lordos EF, Trombert V, Vogt N, et al. Antiepileptic drugs in the treatment of neuropathic pain: drug-to-drug interaction in elderly people. J Am Geriatr Soc 2009; 57(1):181–2.
45. Pino Maria. Trigeminal neuralgia: a "Lightning Bolt" of pain. Available at: https://www.uspharmacist.com/article/trigeminal-neuralgia-a-lightning-bolt-of-pain. Accessed September 7, 2020.

46. Franklin GM. Opioids for chronic noncancer pain: a position paper of the American Academy of Neurology. Neurology 2014;83(14):1277–84.

47. McNicol ED, Midbari A, Eisenberg E. Opioids for neuropathic pain. Cochrane Database Syst Rev 2013;8. https://doi.org/10.1002/14651858.CD006146.pub2.

48. Ali A, Arif AW, Bhan C, et al. Managing chronic pain in the elderly: an Overview of the recent therapeutic Advancements. Cureus 2018;10(9):e3293.

49. Khdour MR. Treatment of diabetic peripheral neuropathy: a review. J Pharm Pharmacol 2020. https://doi.org/10.1111/jphp.13241.

50. Duehmke RM, Derry S, Wiffen PJ, et al. Tramadol for neuropathic pain in adults. Cochrane Database Syst Rev 2017;(6):CD003726.

51. Mijnhout GS, Kollen BJ, Alkhalaf A, et al. Alpha lipoic Acid for symptomatic peripheral neuropathy in patients with diabetes: a meta-analysis of randomized controlled trials. Int J Endocrinol 2012;2012:456279.

52. Ziegler D, Ametov A, Barinov A, et al. Oral treatment with alpha-lipoic acid improves symptomatic diabetic polyneuropathy: the SYDNEY 2 trial. Diabetes Care 2006;29(11):2365–70.

53. El-Nahas MR, Elkannishy G, Abdelhafez H, et al. Oral alpha lipoic acid treatment for symptomatic diabetic peripheral neuropathy: a randomized double-blinded placebo-controlled study. Endocr Metab Immune Disord Drug Targets 2020. https://doi.org/10.2174/1871530320666200506081407.

54. Baicus C, Purcarea A, von Elm E, et al. Alpha-lipoic acid for diabetic peripheral neuropathy. Cochrane Database Syst Rev 2018;2018(2). https://doi.org/10.1002/14651858.CD012967.

55. Pickering G, Lucchini C. Topical treatment of localized neuropathic pain in the elderly. Drugs Aging 2020;37(2):83–9.

56. Pickering G, Martin E, Tiberghien F, et al. Localized neuropathic pain: an expert consensus on local treatments. Drug Des Devel Ther 2017;11:2709–18.

57. Derry S, Wiffen PJ, Moore RA, et al. Topical lidocaine for neuropathic pain in adults. Cochrane Database Syst Rev 2014;7:CD010958.

58. Baron R, Mayoral V, Leijon G, et al. Efficacy and safety of combination therapy with 5% lidocaine medicated plaster and pregabalin in post-herpetic neuralgia and diabetic polyneuropathy. Curr Med Res Opin 2009;25(7):1677–87.

59. Derry S, Rice AS, Cole P, et al. Topical capsaicin (high concentration) for chronic neuropathic pain in adults. Cochrane Database Syst Rev 2017;1. https://doi.org/10.1002/14651858.CD007393.pub4.

60. Haanpää M, Cruccu G, Nurmikko TJ, et al. Capsaicin 8% patch versus oral pregabalin in patients with peripheral neuropathic pain. Eur J Pain Lond Engl 2016;20(2):316–28.

61. Simpson DM, Robinson-Papp J, Van J, et al. Capsaicin 8% patch in painful diabetic peripheral neuropathy: a randomized, double-blind, placebo-controlled study. J Pain 2017;18(1):42–53.

62. Singleton JR, Marcus RL, Lessard M, et al. Supervised exercise improves cutaneous reinnervation capacity in metabolic syndrome patients. Ann Neurol 2015;77(1):146–53.

63. Smith AG, Russell J, Feldman EL, et al. Lifestyle intervention for Pre-diabetic neuropathy. Diabetes Care 2006;29(6):1294–9.

64. Jones RCW, Lawson E, Backonja M. Managing neuropathic pain. Med Clin North Am 2016;100(1):151–67.

65. Ahn S, Song R. Effects of Tai Chi exercise on glucose control, neuropathy scores, balance, and quality of life in patients with type 2 diabetes and neuropathy. J Altern Complement Med 2012;18(12):1172–8.

66. Hung J-W, Liou C-W, Wang P-W, et al. Effect of 12-week tai chi chuan exercise on peripheral nerve modulation in patients with type 2 diabetes mellitus. J Rehabil Med 2009;41(11):924–9.
67. Mooventhan A, Nivethitha L. Evidence based effects of yoga in neurological disorders. J Clin Neurosci 2017;43:61–7.
68. Rowin J. Integrative neuromuscular medicine: neuropathy and neuropathic pain: consider the alternatives. Muscle Nerve 2019;60(2):124–36.
69. Garfinkel MS, Singhal A, Katz WA, et al. Yoga-based intervention for carpal tunnel syndrome: a randomized trial. JAMA 1998;280(18):1601–3.
70. Evans S, Fishman B, Spielman L, et al. Randomized trial of cognitive behavior therapy versus supportive Psychotherapy for HIV-related peripheral neuropathic pain. Psychosomatics 2003;44(1):44–50.
71. Eccleston C, Hearn L, Williams AC de C. Psychological therapies for the management of chronic neuropathic pain in adults. Cochrane Database Syst Rev 2015;10:CD011259.
72. McBeth J, Prescott G, Scotland G, et al. Cognitive behavior therapy, exercise, or both for treating chronic widespread pain. Arch Intern Med 2012;172(1):48–57.
73. Dorfman D, George MC, Schnur J, et al. Hypnosis for treatment of HIV neuropathic pain: a preliminary report. Pain Med Malden Mass 2013;14(7):1048–56.
74. Hussain N, Said ASA. Mindfulness-based meditation versus progressive relaxation meditation: impact on chronic pain in older Female patients with diabetic neuropathy. J Evid-based Integr Med 2019;24. 2515690X19876599.
75. Izgu N, Gok Metin Z, Karadas C, et al. Progressive muscle relaxation and mindfulness meditation on neuropathic pain, fatigue, and quality of life in patients with type 2 diabetes: a randomized clinical trial. J Nurs Scholarsh 2020. https://doi.org/10.1111/jnu.12580.
76. Tavee J, Rensel M, Planchon SM, et al. Effects of meditation on pain and quality of life in multiple sclerosis and peripheral neuropathy: a pilot study. Int J MS Care 2011;13(4):163–8.
77. Teixeira E. The effect of mindfulness meditation on painful diabetic peripheral neuropathy in adults older than 50 years. Holist Nurs Pract 2010;24(5):277–83.
78. Dimitrova A, Murchison C, Oken B. Acupuncture for the treatment of peripheral neuropathy: a systematic review and meta-analysis. J Altern Complement Med N Y N 2017;23(3):164–79.
79. Ju ZY, Wang K, Cui HS, et al. Acupuncture for neuropathic pain in adults. Cochrane Database Syst Rev 2017;(12):CD012057.
80. Mücke M, Phillips T, Radbruch L, et al. Cannabis-based medicines for chronic neuropathic pain in adults. Cochrane Database Syst Rev 2018;3. https://doi.org/10.1002/14651858.CD012182.pub2.
81. Wallace MS, Marcotte TD, Umlauf A, et al. Efficacy of inhaled cannabis on painful diabetic neuropathy. J Pain 2015;16(7):616–27.

Moving?

Make sure your subscription moves with you!

To notify us of your new address, find your **Clinics Account Number** (located on your mailing label above your name), and contact customer service at:

Email: journalscustomerservice-usa@elsevier.com

800-654-2452 (subscribers in the U.S. & Canada)
314-447-8871 (subscribers outside of the U.S. & Canada)

Fax number: 314-447-8029

Elsevier Health Sciences Division
Subscription Customer Service
3251 Riverport Lane
Maryland Heights, MO 63043

*To ensure uninterrupted delivery of your subscription, please notify us at least 4 weeks in advance of move.